CANCER TODAY
Origins, Prevention, and Treatment

Written by Leslie Roberts
Foreword by Lewis Thomas, M.D.

INSTITUTE OF MEDICINE / NATIONAL ACADEMY PRESS
Washington, D.C. 1984

National Academy of Sciences • 2101 Constitution Avenue, NW • Washington, DC 20418

This publication is based on presentations at the annual meeting of the Institute of Medicine held in Washington, D.C. on 26 October 1983. The views expressed are those of the participants and do not necessarily reflect those of the Institute of Medicine.

The Institute of Medicine was chartered in 1970 by the National Academy of Sciences to enlist distinguished members of appropriate professions in the examination of policy matters pertaining to the health of the public. In this, the Institute acts under both the Academy's 1863 congressional charter responsibility to be an adviser to the federal government, and its own initiative in identifying issues of medical care, research, and education.

Library of Congress Cataloging in Publication Data

Roberts, Leslie, 1950-
Cancer today.

Contains summarized report of the 1983 Institute of Medicine Annual Meeting, held in Washington, D.C.
Includes index.
1. Cancer—Congr[redacted]). Meeting (1983: Washington, D.C.) II. Titl[redacted]200 R645c]
RC261.A2R6 1984 6[redacted]

ISBN 0-309-03436-1

Printed in the United States of America

Preface and Acknowledgments

Of all the afflictions of humankind, cancer inspires a particular dread. Perhaps because it carries a tradition of hopelessness that is not dispelled even by new reports of better cure rates, cancer seems to pose a mystery that defies our otherwise remarkable scientific skills.

In truth, however, we have never been closer to understanding exactly how cancer gets its start. This promise carries with it the increasingly good prospect that in a large number of cases the disease can be prevented and possibly cured completely.

To provide a forum on today's optimism about cancer, the Institute of Medicine devoted its 1983 annual meeting to an examination of the scientific advances underlying that optimism. The program, "Implications of New Developments in Science: Cancer," presented some of the newest discoveries in tumor biology, evidence linking diet to cancer, and aspects of treatment and care.

This book, prepared by science writer Leslie Roberts, is based on the presentations given at the 1983 meeting. The chapters on the biology of cancer derive from the talks of J. Michael Bishop,

Philip Leder, and Mariano Barbacid. Anthony Miller, Bruce Ames, and Richard Merrill contributed the bases for the chapters on diet and cancer. Emil Frei, Jimmie Holland, and David Greer provided material for the chapters on chemotherapy, psychosocial aspects of cancer, and American hospices. Finally, the summarizing comments of Paul Marks and Maureen Henderson set the framework for the book's introduction. For the readers' convenience, the back of the book contains a glossary of terms frequently used in the areas of cancer research discussed here.

The Institute of Medicine wishes to thank all the speakers who addressed the 1983 meeting—a complete list follows—for their cooperation throughout the preparation of this book, and to express special gratitude to Lewis Thomas for the foreword, crafted with the grace characteristic of all his writings. We also are very grateful to division director Enriqueta Bond for her guidance in planning and implementing last year's annual meeting.

Cancer Today is an experiment, a new form for communicating the current interests of the Institute of Medicine to the public. We hope for its successful reception and for future opportunities to share our work with a wider audience.

Frederick C. Robbins, M.D.
President, Institute of Medicine

Contents

Participants vi
Foreword vii
Lewis Thomas

1. Introduction 1

Biology of Cancer

2. Genes Gone Awry 17
3. Oncogenes in Human Cancer 29
4. Broken Chromosomes 39

Diet and Cancer

5. The Epidemiology of Diet and Cancer 49
6. Dietary Carcinogens and Anticarcinogens 63
7. Diet and Cancer: New Policy Questions 73

Cancer Treatment

8. Cancer Medicine: Chemotherapy 81
9. The Psychological and Social Effects of Cancer 91
10. Alternative Care for the Dying: American Hospices 103

Glossary 117
Index 121

Participants

MAUREEN HENDERSON, *Meeting Chairman*, Professor of Epidemiology and Medicine, University of Washington

BRUCE N. AMES, Professor of Biochemistry, University of California-Berkeley

MARIANO BARBACID, Head, Developmental Oncology Section, National Cancer Institute-Frederick Cancer Research Facility

J. MICHAEL BISHOP, Professor of Microbiology and Immunology, University of California-San Francisco

EMIL FREI III, Director and Physician-in-Chief, Dana-Farber Cancer Institute

DAVID S. GREER, Dean of Medicine, Professor of Community Health, Brown University

JIMMIE C. HOLLAND, Chief, Psychiatry Service, Memorial Sloan-Kettering Cancer Center

PHILIP LEDER, John Emory Andrus Professor and Chairman, Department of Genetics, Harvard University School of Medicine

PAUL A. MARKS, President, Memorial Sloan-Kettering Cancer Center

RICHARD A. MERRILL, Dean and Professor, School of Law, University of Virginia

ANTHONY B. MILLER, Director, National Cancer Institute of Canada Epidemiologic Unit, University of Toronto

Staff

ENRIQUETA C. BOND, Director, Division of Health Promotion and Disease Prevention, Institute of Medicine

Foreword

There was a time within easy memory when cancer was regarded within the upper circles of basic biomedical science as an unapproachable and therefore not very interesting research problem. Twenty years ago it was generally viewed as an essentially unsolvable puzzle, too profound and complex to be attacked by any imaginable research technology, simply beyond the reach of science.

Not to say that excellent research was not going on. It was, and indeed the groundwork was then being laid by the molecular biochemists, virologists, immunologists, and cell biologists for what was to follow. But at that time, in the 1960s, the cancer problem had not yet engaged the full force of intellectual attention in biomedical science at large, as is the case today. It was not yet perceived that there could be ways into the very depths of the problem. The time, it was said, was not at hand.

In the early 1970s the magnitude of the problem as a cause of incapacitation and death in human beings was recognized as an increasingly serious matter, and pressures were brought on and by the Washington administration and Congress to do something much more ambitious in the way of research. Advisory committees and panels went to work, putting together what soon emerged as the "Conquest of Cancer" plan, backed by the assurance of greatly expanded budgets for cancer research. The arguments over how to go about it were intense and sometimes bitter. Some of the scientific advisers asserted that it was just too early for a full-scale attack; too much fundamental information was lacking. Others believed that the country should invest heavily in applied science, in an endeavor to improve what already existed in therapeutic, diagnostic, and preventive medicine.

This was, as it turned out, one of the luckier turning points in the history of biomedical science and the inevitable politics associated with science. Two things happened at about the same time. Research funds became available on a scale to attract many investigators, especially the youngest and brightest, into a field that they might otherwise not have chosen to enter. This in itself was an important event, but if it had occurred by itself we would not find ourselves where we are in the mid-1980s. Money is of course crucial for the progress of science, but money alone cannot make science.

Science makes itself, grows itself, and is transformed by its own upheavals and surprises, and this is what began to happen, quite coincidentally and spontaneously, at just the time when the new cancer research program was launched. The biological revolution, as it was then termed, which had begun with the discovery that DNA was the essential genetic material, possessing a molecular structure to account nicely for replication and duplication, was suddenly transformed into a new revolution superimposed on the old one. First came the discovery of cellular enzymes specifically designed to clip segments of DNA at predictable sites along the molecule, and at the same time an array of vastly improved instrumentation techniques for sequencing the molecular fragments, and finally, like a burst of drums, the brand new, unpredicted and astonishing technology of recombinant DNA. Cancer had become, almost overnight, a new kind of adventure for the cell biologists, experimental pathologists, virologists, immunologists, and geneticists, and it moved to the center of biomedical science as the most fascinating and engaging of puzzles.

And so it is today. The recombinant DNA technology, surely the most important scientific advance of the century in biology, was soon reinforced and supplemented by the invention of hybridomas and the elaboration of monoclonal antibodies, now indispensable for the identification of gene products and surface markers in transformed cells.

The role of oncogenes and their mobile geometric localization at different sites within the genome, the existence of enhancing genes and the crucial role of their location in relation to oncogenes, the mode of action of cancer viruses, the complex defense mechanisms mediated and modulated by the various T-lymphocyte populations—all these and more breakthroughs still to come have changed everything about the cancer problem.

I have never known a time of such high confidence and exhilaration within the community of biomedical scientists, especially among the youngest investigators just coming on the scene at the postdoctoral level. Cancer research has turned into something like a running hunt. The fox is not yet within sight, but it is at least known that there is indeed a fox, and this is a great change from the sense of things twenty years ago. At that time it was generally believed that cancer was not one disease but a hundred, all fundamentally different and each requiring its own unique penetration. Today it seems much more likely that a single mechanism, or a set of mechanisms, lurks at the deep center of every form of cancer. It is even conceivable, in this writer's optimistic view, that when all the facts are in there may emerge a totally new, still unpredictable combination of applied pharmacology and immunology for reversal of the process and for its prevention.

The way ahead is now open for the clinical scientists and epidemiologists to begin asking questions, unthinkable a generation back, about the role of environmental factors, including nutrition, in the causation of cancer. Very likely, the rising generation of oncology investigators will become even more dependent on experimental animal models for answers, but *in vitro* cell culture systems will also have more to offer than ever before.

The book before you is a brief but comprehensive summary—an overview—of where things stand today in cancer research. If the work goes on at its present pace, some things will change next week or next month, and everything may look quite different next year. But the drift of events laid out in the chapters of this volume should convey a sense of the ways in which progress has been made up to now, and also some sense, cautious as it should be, of the hopes for the future.

Lewis Thomas, M.D.
President Emeritus, Memorial
Sloan-Kettering Cancer Center

CANCER TODAY

1

Introduction

There is a new sense of optimism pervading cancer hospitals and research laboratories. Scientific advances of the past few decades have brought steady increases in the cancer survival rate. It is estimated that nearly 50 percent of all patients diagnosed with cancer in 1984 will be cured (see Figures 1-1, 1-2). A decade ago, the figure was 40 percent.

New techniques have been found for early detection and diagnosis; new therapies are becoming available for treating some of the highly recalcitrant forms of cancer. And in the past few years, molecular biologists have begun to understand the fundamental nature of the cancer cell. Their work promises to reveal how the disease gets started in its many forms, opening up new possibilities for prevention and treatment. This book describes the

---

This chapter is based on the remarks of Maureen Henderson, University of Washington, and Paul A. Marks, Memorial Sloan-Kettering Cancer Center, at the 1983 annual meeting of the Institute of Medicine. Dr. Henderson served as chairman of the meeting.

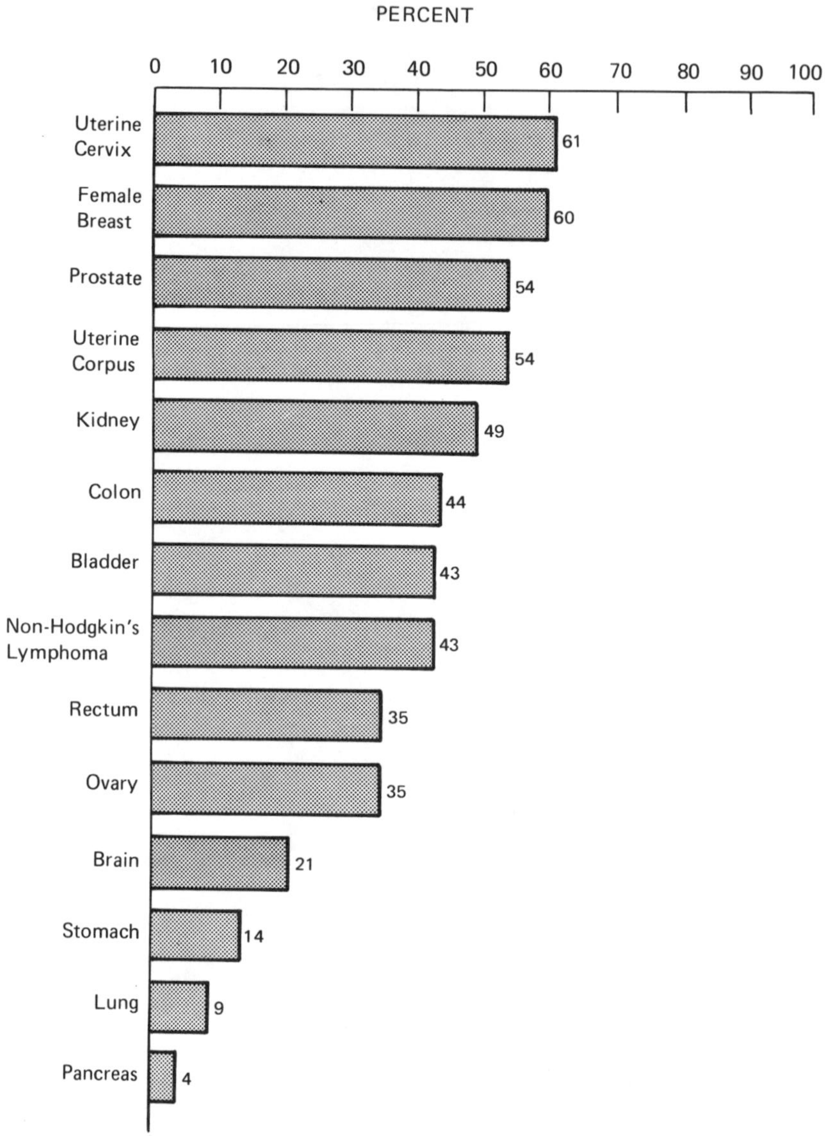

FIGURE 1–1 Five-year relative survival rates for black patients, 1973–1979. (*Source:* SEER Program, National Cancer Institute, 1983.)

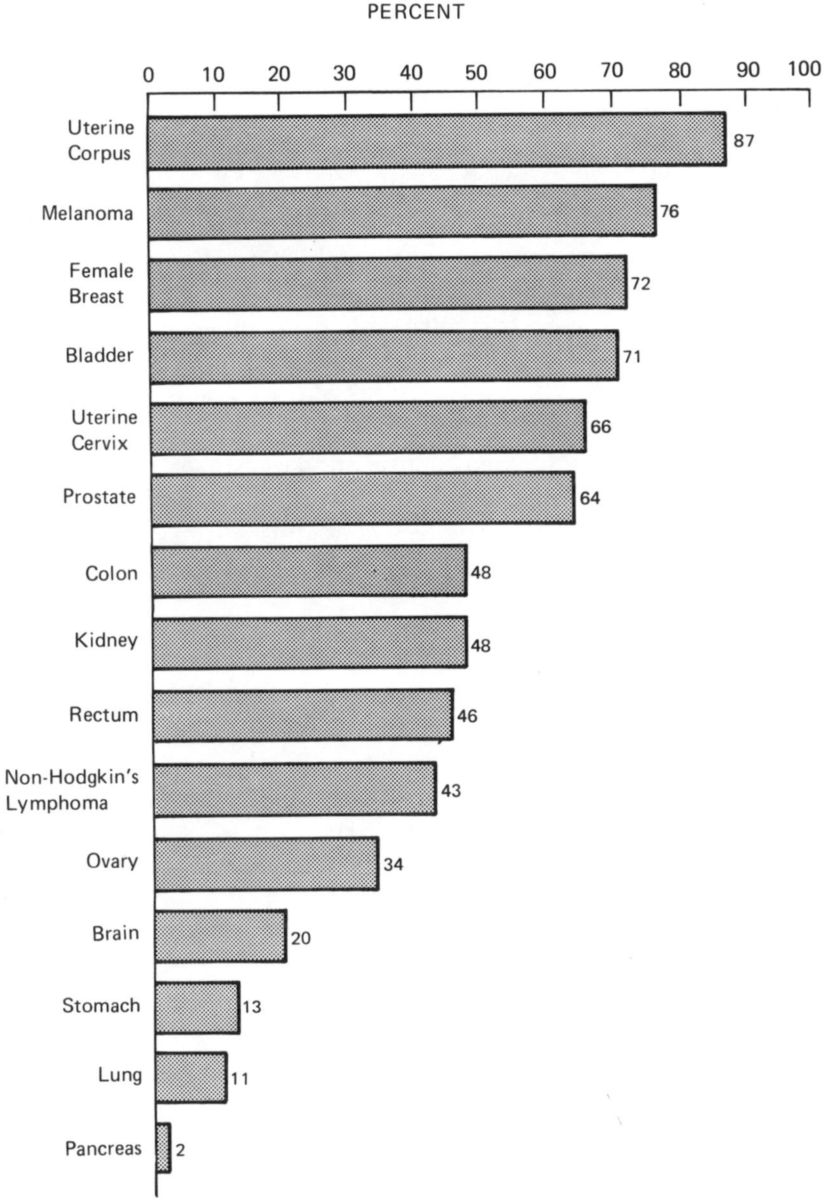

FIGURE 1–2 Five-year relative survival rates for white patients, 1973–1979. (*Source:* SEER Program, National Cancer Institute, 1983.)

continuing efforts of researchers in a broad spectrum of disciplines to understand and control cancer.

Cancer is still a disease of tragic dimensions. One of every four Americans will develop cancer and one in five will die of it, if current incidence and mortality rates remain the same. It is the second largest cause of death in this country, exceeded only by heart disease. In 1984, there will be 870,000 new cases of cancer and 450,000 cancer deaths, approximately 20 percent of all deaths this year (see Table 1-1).

Half of all cancer deaths will result from malignancies of the lung, colon and rectum, breast, and pancreas. Lung cancer, which is closely tied to tobacco consumption, alone accounts for over 20 percent of all cancer deaths. Among men, it is the largest cause of cancer death; among women, the second largest (see Figure 1-3).

Although the incidence and mortality rates for lung cancer have soared during the last 50 years, the age-adjusted rates for cancers at most other sites have remained steady or declined.[1] For some

TABLE 1–1 Estimated New Cases and Deaths for Major Sites of Cancer—1984*

Site	No. of Cases	Deaths
Lung	139,000	121,000
Colon-Rectum	130,000	59,000
Breast	116,000	38,000
Prostate	76,000	25,000
Uterus	55,000**	10,000
Urinary	57,000	19,000
Oral	27,000	9,000
Pancreas	25,000	23,000
Leukemia	24,000	17,000
Ovary	18,000	12,000
Skin	18,000***	7,000

*Figures rounded to nearest 1,000.
**If carcinoma in situ is included, cases total over 99,000.
***Estimated new cases of nonmelanoma about 400,000.

(SOURCE: American Cancer Society, *Cancer Facts and Figures 1984*.)

[1] The actual number of people who develop and die of cancer has increased throughout this period, largely because a major segment of the population is reaching the age when cancers usually develop.

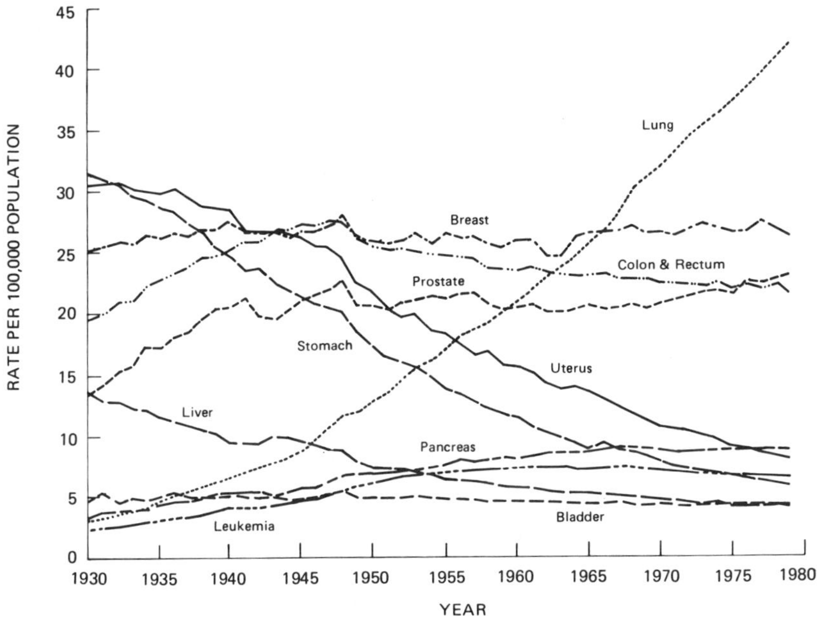

FIGURE 1–3 Age-adjusted cancer death rates by site, United States, 1930–1979. (*SOURCE:* American Cancer Society, *Cancer Facts and Figures 1984*.)

cancers, this reflects a drop in the incidence, or the number of new cancer cases; for others, the striking improvements in the cure rate for certain cancers.

Cancer takes many forms, striking different types of cells in diverse parts of the body. Each cancer runs its own distinctive course. For instance, although cancer usually appears as a tumor—a visible mass of cancer cells—in leukemia the malignant cells largely remain dispersed throughout the body in the blood and bone marrow.

All of these cancers, however, share the same fundamental properties. Cancer is a breakdown of the orderly process of cell growth and differentiation. It seems to begin with a change in a single cell, presumably a mutation in that cell's genetic apparatus. This change transforms the cell profoundly; it begins to divide without restraint, failing to differentiate into its mature form. Eventually, this altered cell will give rise to billions of other aberrant cells, cancer cells, that invade and destroy nearby tissues. As the colony grows, some of these cells will break off, or metastasize, and be carried by the blood or lymph stream to remote parts of the body where they will invade other tissues as well.

The first section of this report describes some of the phenomenal strides of the past decade in determining the biological basis of cancer. Specifically, it recounts the discovery of cancer genes and the preliminary insights this research has provided into the genetic and biochemical changes that give rise to cancer.

On another front, researchers have been seeking the external factors that cause or contribute to cancer. The role of some agents, including radiation, certain occupational or environmental chemicals, and tobacco, are well documented. New studies discussed in the second section suggest that diet and nutrition may also be responsible for a significant portion—as much as 30 percent—of all cancers in the United States, which opens up new possibilities for prevention.

The work under way in molecular biology laboratories here and abroad promises to profoundly alter approaches to cancer treatment and prevention. In the near term, however, the major advances in cancer survival will probably come from improvements in conventional cancer drugs developed over the past three decades, according to Paul A. Marks, president of Memorial Sloan-Kettering Cancer Center. Eventually, the recent discoveries in molecular biology should contribute to the development of a whole new order of chemotherapeutic agents. The final section of this report describes progress and potential in the treatment of cancer, as well as new approaches to ameliorating the devastating psychological effects of the disease.

The Biology of Cancer

In the early 1970s, cancer research was galvanized by the discovery of oncogenes, specific genes that can trigger a cell's unbridled growth. Since that time, close to 30 of these cancer genes have been isolated from both human and animal cells. In laboratory experiments, the activity of a single one of them is often sufficient to transform normal cells to cancer cells.

In the past few years, molecular biologists have been able to decipher the genetic code of these cancer genes. To their surprise, they found that the oncogenes are remarkably similar, if not identical, to benign genes that are normally present within the cell. It now appears that each cell contains certain normal genes that when activated or altered in some way can start the cell on the path to cancer. Many cancer researchers suspect that all agents of cancer—radiation, chemicals, and viruses—act upon these genes, somehow releasing their malignant potential.

Investigators have already identified several mechanisms that activate these genes, transforming them from an innocuous to a malignant state. More such mechanisms will undoubtedly be discovered. One of the greatest challenges to cancer biologists in the coming years will be to determine how the oncogenes differ from normal genes, and where and how they act in the cell to induce cancer.

Like other genes, an oncogene directs the synthesis of a protein, which in turn performs some specific biochemical activity within the cell. The key to understanding cancer would seem to lie in these oncogene proteins, for it is their activity that renders the cell malignant. In the past few years, molecular biologists have begun to identify and study some of these cancer proteins, gaining the first glimpses into the biochemical activities that induce cancer. The evidence to date is tantalizing: it suggests that cancer may arise from a very subtle distortion of normal cellular processes.

This work is just beginning; many questions remain. It is still not clear whether oncogenes are involved in all or just some cancers. Nor is it known how they fit into the overall scheme of carcinogenesis, which in humans is a complex process involving many discrete steps and often taking 20 years. While the activation of an oncogene may be a necessary part of this process, it is not sufficent to induce human cancer.

If the past few years are any indication, answers to some of these questions may be available in the coming months and years. It is impossible to predict, however, which lines of research will prove the most fruitful. The discoveries that have revealed oncogenes to date have come from a convergence of some surprisingly disparate research pursuits.

Investigators were led to human oncogenes by the study of tumor viruses found in experimental animals. Many of the insights into the activation and function of these genes have come from yet other fields. For instance, some 30 years ago Barbara McClintock first proposed that genes are not static or permanently fixed on the chromosome. Rather, her studies of the corn plant suggested that genes might be capable of moving from place to place on the same chromosome, or even of jumping from chromosome to chromosome, thereby altering the expression of nearby genes. Over the past few years, some basic researchers studying the genetics of the human immune system have revealed how McClintock's process of DNA rearrangement might serve to activate an oncogene, at least in one type of cancer.

Although McClintock and others were doing work relevant to understanding cancer decades ago, the technology needed to confirm their ideas and tie them to the disease process has been available only for the past 10 years or so. Without recombinant DNA and other genetic technologies, most recent research in molecular biology could not have proceeded. It is these technologies that have enabled researchers for the first time to isolate and study a single gene from among the tens of thousands contained in a human cell.

The next three chapters of this report describe the discovery of oncogenes and the continuing efforts to determine their function. For those readers who do not choose to dwell long on the intricacies of cancer genes, Chapter 2 should suffice to convey both the excitement and the potential of this new field. For those who want a more detailed understanding of the molecular basis of cancer, Chapters 3 and 4 attempt to provide it in accessible language.

Diet and Cancer

Even before the discovery of oncogenes, it was thought that cancer, at least in some of its manifestations, was the product of the interaction of genes and the environment. Certain agents, such as ultraviolet and ionizing radiation, some chemicals, and some viruses, can initiate cancer, presumably by causing a genetic mutation. From recent work, it is tempting to think that the mutation occurs on an oncogene. Still other external or environmental agents can promote or facilitate the process of carcinogenesis without actually inducing it.

There is now widespread agreement that roughly 85 percent of all cancers are caused by broad environmental factors, including lifestyle patterns. The rest, presumably, have a hereditary basis, or else arise from spontaneous metabolic events. Identifying the environmental factors in cancer, however, has not been easy. At this stage, viruses appear to play only a minor role in human cancers. Occupational chemicals are thought to be responsible for 4 percent of all cancers; environmental chemicals for an estimated 2 percent. Tobacco is by far the largest documented cause of cancer, accounting for roughly 30 percent of all cancers in lungs and some other sites.

Recently, epidemiological studies similar to those that uncovered an association between smoking and cancer have detected a link between the foods that people eat and the cancers that afflict them. Overall, dietary factors are thought to be responsible for another 30 percent of the cancer incidence in the United States, which could mean that a substantial portion of those cancers may be preventable.

With a few exceptions, the studies have not turned up specific culprits—certain foods or constitutents of foods that cause cancer. Nor does the major problem appear to be food additives or contaminants. Rather, as described in Chapter 5, cancer risk is associated with certain broad dietary patterns and the consumption of major nutrients. Specifically, a diet high in fats and fatty meats seems to carry a risk of cancer. Salt-cured, salt-pickled, and highly spiced foods are also suspect. On the other hand, the consumption of high-fiber grains, vegetables, and fruits seems to protect against cancer. In short, cancer risk appears to be a matter of dietary choice, of the balance and proportion of nutrients in the diet, as well as of methods of food preparation.

The case against diet is still circumstantial. These epidemiological studies have revealed broad associations, not causality. Further laboratory and clinical studies are necessary to determine exactly how diet contributes to cancer. For instance, the specific dietary constituents that may be responsible for observed carcinogenic or protective effects are not known, nor are their mechanisms of action. Nonetheless, several federal agencies have decided that the weight of evidence is strong enough to suggest that the public modify its eating habits in accordance with the findings of these studies.

This is not to imply that a modification in diet would elicit a reduction in cancer incidence similar to the one that would result if smoking were eliminated. Studies to date have made it abundantly clear that the relationship of diet to cancer is exceedingly complex. The risk factors in diet cannot simply be eliminated; some of the dietary constitutents that seem to pose greatest cancer risk are essential human nutrients.

In addition, as described in Chapter 6, it has become increasingly clear from another line of inquiry that natural mutagens and carcinogens are ubiquitous throughout the human diet, occurring in common vegetables, fruits, meats, nuts, and beverages. Conversely, some natural substances, such as the precursor of vitamin A and the mineral selenium, appear to be anticarcinogens, capable of preventing the process of malignant transformation in laboratory studies.

At this stage, the potency of most of the natural carcinogens and the magnitude of risk they pose to human health have not been determined, nor is it known if and how they might interact with anticarcinogens in the diet. What does seem clear, however, is that it will not be possible to specify a risk-free diet.

Cancer researchers generally agree that adoption of a low-risk diet should help to prevent some cancers. The exact benefit to be gained, however, cannot be predicted until the biological mechanisms underlying the association between diet and cancer are better understood.

Chapter 7 discusses the implications of these new findings for the federal approach to cancer prevention. Traditionally, the government has acted through its regulatory policies to minimize human exposure to harmful substances in foods. It has set standards for food additives and natural contaminants, as well as for pesticide residues and other industrial chemicals that might enter the food supply. Now that foods themselves, not the substances added to them, appear to pose the greatest cancer risk, this regulatory approach no longer appears sufficient, although it is certainly a vital element of any food safety policy. Indeed, the most effective strategy for preventing cancer may simply be to provide information that will help consumers make intelligent dietary decisions, giving them an increasing share of the responsibility for their own protection.

Cancer Medicine

The impressive gains in cancer survival of the past three decades stem in large part from advances in chemotherapy. When the effort to develop cancer drugs and appropriate therapeutic regimens began in the 1940s, investigators had few clues into the nature of carcinogenesis and thus little rational basis for testing one compound over another. Trial and error played a substantial part in early chemotherapy research, as described in Chapter 8. From 1955 to 1975, some 40,000 compounds were screened each year in hope of finding a few capable of killing cancer cells. Once those compounds were detected, clinical investigators tried them in various doses and combinations until they found the most effective regimen.

Some 30 chemotherapeutic agents are now available, most of them developed beween 1940 and 1965. Their use has brought a dramatic reversal in the prognosis for some types of cancer. For instance, in 1955 virtually every child afflicted with acute lymphocytic leukemia died of the disease, usually within a few months of diagnosis. Today the cure rate is 58 percent.

Despite these dramatic successes, chemotherapy has several limitations. One is the ease with which cancer cells can become resistant to many of these drugs, rendering them ineffective. Another is the extreme toxicity of certain cancer drugs. Chemotherapeutic agents work by killing cancer cells, and they invariably kill some normal cells as well. The cells in the intestinal mucosa, bone marrow, and hair follicles are the most vulnerable to attack, which explains the common side effects of nausea, vomiting, and hair loss.

Perhaps more important, none of the existing agents is totally effective against the most prevalent form of cancer, the carcinomas, or malignancies of the epithelial tissues, which develop in the head, neck, breast, lung, bowel, and other organs.

The search for new antitumor agents is continuing, as are efforts to increase the effectiveness or reduce the side effects of existing drugs. For the future, advances in molecular biology—both in the understanding of the nature of cancerous transformation and in the refinement of genetic engineering techniques—offer novel approaches to chemotherapy.

As mentioned earlier, toxicity is a problem because it has not been possible to target a cytotoxic drug exclusively to cancer cells. The new genetic technologies may change that. Tumor cells bear distinctive antigens, or proteins, on their surface. Investigators are now trying to develop very specific antibodies, known as monoclonal antibodies, that will interact with only those tumor antigens. Conceivably, these antibodies could be used to deliver a cancer drug to that cell and that cell alone.

Genetic technologies may also provide methods of arresting cancer without relying on cytotoxic drugs. One approach under study would enlist the aid of some of the substances, such as interferon and growth factors, that cells produce to regulate their growth and provide defense against disease. It may also be possible to manipulate the immune system so that it is better able to fight off cancer. Eventually, it may even prove feasible to turn off oncogenes and halt the process of carcinogenesis, or perhaps to somehow interfere with the oncogene protein product.

Early Detection

The chances of successful treatment are greatly enhanced if the cancer is discovered at an early stage, before it has invaded adjacent tissues. One factor in the increasing cure rate has been the introduction of techniques for the early detection of cancer. For instance, the widespread adoption of the "Pap smear" has been credited with a 50 percent decline in the death rate from cervical cancer in the United States. According to Paul Marks, new techniques for diagnosing tumors at early stages may offer the greatest near-term potential for improving the ability to treat common cancers.

Researchers are now studying techniques to enable the detection of minute tumors and even microscopic metastases in inaccessible parts of the body. Although this work is not covered in this report, it deserves mention here because of its vast potential for improving cancer treatment and survival. Such techniques would be useful not only in the early detection of cancer, but also as diagnostic devices to determine how far the cancer has spread, or to monitor the patient's response to therapy and warn of any recurrence at an early stage.

Genetic engineering technology makes possible the large-scale production of specific cancer antibodies, which can also be used in diagnosis. Labeled with a radioactive tag, these antibodies can search out minute tumors or dispersed cancer cells.

The new imaging techniques also show considerable promise for detecting tumors in inaccessible sites. The CAT scan, or computerized axial tomograph, involves the use of a computer to reconstruct X-ray data into images of plane sections of the body. Nuclear magnetic resonance, or NMR, which uses magnetic fields to produce a cross-sectional image of the body, has the added advantage of sparing the patient exposure to potentially harmful X rays.

The Psychological Effects of Cancer

Until recently, most clinical research has focused on methods to detect and treat cancer—surgery to cut away the tumor, drugs and radiation to shrink or destroy it. Yet there has also been a growing realization that to effectively treat cancer, the clinician must understand not only the physical course of the disease, but its effects on the psyche as well. The past decade has seen the emergence of psychosocial research on cancer care, which seeks to understand and mitigate the psychological and social consequences of cancer (Chapter 9).

Investigators have found, for example, that advances in cancer treatment have spawned an entirely new set of issues, those of the cured cancer patient. These cancer survivors, as they are called, face medical, psychological, and social problems during the transition back to an active, healthy life. For one, their future health is uncertain: they are at risk of developing a secondary malignancy or they may suffer consequences from chemotherapy or radiation therapy, such as damage to reproductive organs. Little is known about the long-term effects of these traumatic therapies. Investigations are now under way to determine the extent of these and other physical problems, as well as the psychological scars that may linger after the symptoms of the disease have disappeared.

Similarly, at some time during or after treatment, all patients experience bouts of emotional turmoil—anger, depression, anxiety, and above all, fear. For some patients, the distress can be debilitating, warranting psychiatric intervention of some kind. Yet all too often the turmoil and depression have been considered an inevitable consequence of cancer, as have the stresses on the family and the medical staff, and little has been done to alleviate them. Psychosocial researchers are now beginning to assess the effectiveness of psychotropic drugs and counseling for cancer patients. Others are studying the psychological and social problems confronting the family and medical staff.

One of the most obvious expressions of the increased concern for the emotional as well as physical well-being of cancer patients is the emergence of the hospice movement in the United States. The first U.S. hospice, a center for treatment of terminally ill patients, was established in 1974; now over 1,000 institutions throughout the country offer hospice care. Hospices focus on emotional support and relief of pain, rather than on intensive, continual medical interventions that may serve to prolong life by a few days or weeks. Families and friends play a major role in patient care; indeed, the patient often remains at home throughout the illness.

The first major study comparing hospice with conventional care is summarized in Chapter 10. This study, mandated by Congress, turned up distinct differences in the type of medical and social services a patient is likely to receive in each system, concluding that each apparently has distinct advantages for certain types of patients.

Implications

For several decades, clinical investigators have been quietly working at improving the lot of the cancer patient. They have developed better diagnostic techniques; drugs with fewer side effects; less disfiguring forms of surgery; safer, more effective uses of radiation; and new types of care for those patients who will ultimately succumb to cancer.

During this time, epidemiologists have identified some of the external factors that cause or contribute to cancer. And most recently, molecular biologists have begun to understand how the disease is initiated within the cell.

The implication of this massive research effort, says Paul Marks, is not that cancer will fade away in the next few years, or even decades. Indeed, he adds, the discovery of oncogenes suggests that cancer may be an integral part of living, the result of the interaction of our genes with the environment. Certainly, an understanding of the fundamental nature of carcinogenesis will transform the nature of clinical care. But it will not yield a magic bullet to cure the disease, nor a vaccine to prevent it. Cancer will not be eradicated like smallpox or polio. Rather, what seems likely to emerge are new approaches to early diagnosis of cancers and new techniques to treat them, providing steady gains in our ability to cure and, more important, to prevent cancer.

2

Genes Gone Awry

Every minute 10 million cells divide in the human body. Usually, they divide in the right way and at the right time, governed by a complex set of controls that have yet to be fully elucidated. When those controls fail, cancer may arise. The carefully ordered pattern of cell growth, division, and differentiation is lost. Instead, the cells begin to divide relentlessly, proliferating and massing into a tumor.

Throughout the course of modern biology, researchers have been trying to determine what causes a cancer cell to run amok. As early as 1866, the French physician Pierre Paul Broca suspected a hereditary basis for the disease. That year he published the lineage of his wife's family, which revealed a clear predisposition to breast cancer. Subsequent investigators also pursued a more general genetic explanation for cancer, reasoning that it must arise from

---

This chapter is based on the presentation given by J. Michael Bishop, University of California-San Francisco, at the 1983 annual meeting of the Institute of Medicine.

damage to DNA, the genetic material, perhaps resulting in a breakdown of the genetic regulation of the cell.

The search apparently has reached its goal. Molecular biologists have found in the chromosomes of both animal and human cells a set of genes that can trigger cancer's unbridled growth. These oncogenes, as they are called, are normal genes that have gone awry. In their benign state, these genes perform some as yet unknown, but certainly essential, function in cell metabolism. Yet when they are inappropriately activated or altered in some way, these genes can start a cell on the path to cancer.

Over two dozen oncogenes have been detected to date in a variety of different types of tumors. The exact way in which these oncogenes participate in the process of cancer remains obscure. Nor is it clear if they are involved in all or only some types of cancer. Investigators are beginning to understand some of the mechanisms that switch on these malignant genes. A far greater challenge will be to determine where and how these genes wreak their havoc in the cell—what proteins they make, and the nature of their function.

The Legacy From Viruses

The current insights into the genetics of cancer stem largely from research on viruses that cause tumors in certain animals. Tumor viruses have been studied sporadically since about 1910, when Francis Peyton Rous identified an infectious agent, which he assumed was a virus, that caused a particular type of cancer, known as a sarcoma, in chickens. Viruses are now known to cause a variety of animal cancers. The notion that viruses also cause human cancer has come in and out of favor since Rous' discovery. Recently, viruses have indeed been detected in some human tumors. This research is continuing, but at this time viruses do not appear to be a major cause of human cancer; thus other mechanisms must be sought.

The most intriguing new findings in cancer biology have come from another line of research on cancer viruses. Rather than probe the causative role of tumor viruses in human cancer, some virologists began in the 1960s to use them as experimental tools to study what goes wrong in a cancer cell. Cancer seems to have many causes, such as radiation, chemicals, and perhaps viruses. Yet in each manifestation, the pattern is the same: the cell becomes disorganized and begins uncontrolled division. This suggests that cancer may proceed through the same molecular mechanisms no matter what its cause. Animal tumor viruses afford a powerful tool to ferret out these mechanisms, for by infecting normal cells with a tumor virus, investigators can observe the process of cancerous transformation in the laboratory.

Retroviruses

Viruses are essentially a packet of genetic information encased in a protein sheath. Researchers have found that many animal tumor viruses, including the sarcoma virus detected by Rous, belong to a family of viruses known as retroviruses. These differ from other viruses and from higher organisms in that their genetic material is not DNA (deoxyribonucleic acid) but the related molecule RNA (ribonucleic acid). Consequently, an extra step is involved in viral replication and gene expression. During the normal course of events in cell growth, the DNA molecules replicate themselves prior to cell division, producing one copy for each eventual daughter cell. The genetic information is expressed when DNA is transcribed into RNA, which then directs the synthesis of the protein encoded by the gene. Thus for retroviruses, RNA first must be reverse transcribed, or copied backward, into DNA, before the virus can replicate or infect a cell. Once this DNA copy has been made, it is inserted into the chromosomal DNA of the host cell that the virus infects. When the host cell DNA then replicates and undergoes transcription into RNA, it expresses the inserted viral genes along with its own genes. As a result, the host animal cell begins to make the proteins coded for by the viral genes, becoming, in essence, a virus factory.

Investigators have found two distinct routes by which retroviruses can induce cancer. One route is insertional mutagenesis: when a retrovirus inserts its DNA into the chromosomal DNA of the host cell, it mutates one or more genes of the host cell in the process. Some of these mutations can engender cancer.

The second route, which came to light in the early 1970s, is through the action of specific cancer-causing genes. One of the key discoveries was made by G. Steven Martin of the University of California at Berkeley, who was studying the Rous sarcoma virus. This is a minute virus, containing only four genes—by contrast, a higher organism has tens of thousands of genes. Through a series of experiments, Martin found that just one gene of the Rous sarcoma virus is responsible for the entire cancerous transformation of a cell. (The other three genes are involved in replication of the virus.) Martin had detected an oncogene. That gene, now known as *src* for the sarcoma, or tumor, it induces, has since been more precisely identified by Peter H. Duesberg of Berkeley and Charles Weissmann, Martin Billeter, and John M. Coffin of the University of Zurich.

Further research revealed that many other retroviruses also carry oncogenes, although some do not. It is this latter group of retroviruses—those without oncogenes—that causes cancer through insertional mutagenesis. It has also recently been learned that these two forms of carcinogenesis are related in an unexpected way, which will be described later.

About twenty retroviral oncogenes have been identified, each with a three-letter name such as *src*, *myc*, and *ras*. All of these genes are able to transform cells in culture, that is, to trigger cancerous growth. Oncogenes, like other genes, direct the synthesis of a specific protein, and it is these oncogene proteins that must be the actual culprits. At this stage, however, researchers have few clues to where and how these proteins act in the cell to induce cancer.

Wayward Genes

Soon after Martin's discovery, an intense research effort began on the oncogenes carried by retroviruses. The hope was that these genes would not turn out to be anomalies related only to a specific type of virally induced cancer, but that they might instead reveal something about the abnormalities of all cancer cells. In this vein, two researchers at the National Cancer Institute (NCI), Robert J. Huebner and George J. Todaro, soon developed the oncogene hypothesis. They postulated that once an oncogene is inserted into an animal or human cell by a virus, it becomes a stable part of that cell's genetic complement, or genome, passed from one generation to the next. It remains a harmless resident of the cell until a carcinogen, such as radiation or a chemical, spurs it to action.

If so, then oncogenes should be present in normal animal cells. J. Michael Bishop, Harold E. Varmus, and Dominique Stehelin of the University of California at San Francisco (UCSF) began looking for them. They soon found the *src* gene in the cells of healthy chickens that had not been infected by a retrovirus. They went on to find a nearly identical gene in every animal tested, from rodents to human beings. It looked as if Huebner and Todaro might be right.

Yet when the UCSF team examined the *src* gene from the healthy chicken cell in detail, they found it was not a viral gene at all, as Huebner and Todaro would have predicted. Instead, it bore the distinctive markings of a vertebrate gene; it was an integral part of the chicken's genome. Moreover, in the healthy cell the gene was active, so it obviously had a different function from its cancer-causing counterpart in the retrovirus. This finding added an unexpected twist to the oncogene hypothesis: it turns out that retroviral oncogenes are actually wayward cellular genes, picked up by the virus during its evolution. Since this initial discovery by Bishop and Varmus, close relatives of all the retroviral oncogenes have been found in normal cells. They are indeed harmless residents, and are called cellular oncogenes, or proto-oncogenes. They are designated c-*src* or c-*myc*, etc., to distinguish them from the viral oncogenes, v-*src* or v-*myc*.

What these proto-oncogenes are doing in the cell is not known, but obviously, as Varmus has said, they were not put there to cause cancer. There are several clues, however. First, these proto-oncogenes have been conserved throughout vertebrate evolution. In other words, the same gene, such as the *src* proto-oncogene or the *myc* proto-oncogene, appears in almost identical form in all types of vertebrates. Some of these genes have even been found in invertebrates, such as fruit flies, and in yeast. That the proto-oncogenes have survived long periods of evolution unchanged indicates that they play an essential, if unknown, role in cell metabolism. And because cancer involves a disruption of normal cellular growth, investigators suspect that proto-oncogenes are involved in the regulation of cell development and differentiation.

The Enemy Within

Retroviral oncogenes, then, appear to be slightly altered versions of normal genes; they are normal cellular genes gone awry. Within the cell, the proto-oncogene is benign. Yet when it is seized by a retrovirus and reintroduced into a cell, its malignant potential is unleashed. In some way as yet unknown, recombination with a retrovirus turns friend into foe.

Experiments by George F. Vande Woude and Edward M. Scolnick of the National Cancer Institute have provided evidence that the normal proto-oncogenes and viral oncogenes are one and the same. The unaltered proto-oncogenes do not transform cells in culture, as do the active, viral oncogenes. Yet when the researchers hooked up each of two proto-oncogenes (*ras* and *mos*) to a piece of viral DNA—a piece that dictates brisk expression of nearby genes—the proto-oncogene was able to convert normal cells to cancer cells.

It is not clear how oncogenes disrupt normal cellular behavior. What is particularly puzzling is that the cancer-causing genes and their normal counterparts appear to be virtually the same. The proteins made by some of the oncogenes and their related proto-oncogenes have recently been identified, and those, too, appear to be quite similar. The question, then, is how to account for the dramatic difference in their functions. Two possible explanations have been proposed. One is that the gene is slightly mutated when it is captured by the virus, resulting in a slightly different protein having abnormal activity. Indeed, all retroviral oncogenes examined to date are clearly damaged or mutated versions of their proto-oncogene precursors. The other explanation is that once the cellular gene is put under viral controls, it is expressed at the wrong time, or in the wrong amount, producing an overabundance of its protein product. Evidence exists for this hypothesis as well. Vande Woude and Scolnick found that when the *ras* and *mos* proto-oncogenes were put under viral control, their expression was enhanced, which suggests that at least in some cases an increased dosage of a normal protein may be involved in the initation of cancerous growth.

Other researchers have found that those retroviruses that do not contain oncogenes—and instead induce cancer through insertional mutagenesis—also act on the normal proto-oncogenes contained in an animal cell. William S. Hayward and Benjamin G. Neel of the Memorial Sloan-Kettering Cancer Center and Susan M. Astrin of the Institute for Cancer Research in Fox Chase, Pennsylvania, have studied the site of insertion for one of these retroviruses, the chicken lymphoma virus. They have found that the viral DNA is almost always inserted into the chicken genome in the immediate vicinity of the *myc* proto-oncogene. Insertion seems to change c-*myc*, for its expression is greatly enhanced. The same has been found for other retroviruses that do not contain their own oncogenes. It appears that these retroviruses exploit the cellular proto-oncogenes to induce tumors.

More recently, activated oncogenes have also been detected in human tumors in which viruses are not involved. From these and other findings, a new cancer theory has emerged. Many biologists now believe that oncogenes lie at the heart of every cancer, no matter what its cause. They suspect that all agents of cancer—viruses, radiation, and chemicals—act upon the family of proto-oncogenes contained in each cell, somehow rendering them malignant (Figure 2-1).

There appear to be many ways to turn on an oncogene. Two have been identified so far in human cancers. Investigators recently found that the oncogene present in human bladder cancer is activated by a mutation in the gene's coding region, that is, where the instructions for making proteins lie. It is the smallest mutation possible (the substitution of a single nucleotide base), yet it is sufficient to instruct the gene to produce a slightly abnormal protein, rather than an overabundance of a normal protein, as has been found in the viral oncogenes. In another human cancer, Burkitt lymphoma, the *myc* oncogene appears to be activated when a chromosome breaks and the gene is plucked from its usual site and inserted into a more active site on another chromosome. These modes of activation will be described in detail in the following two chapters.

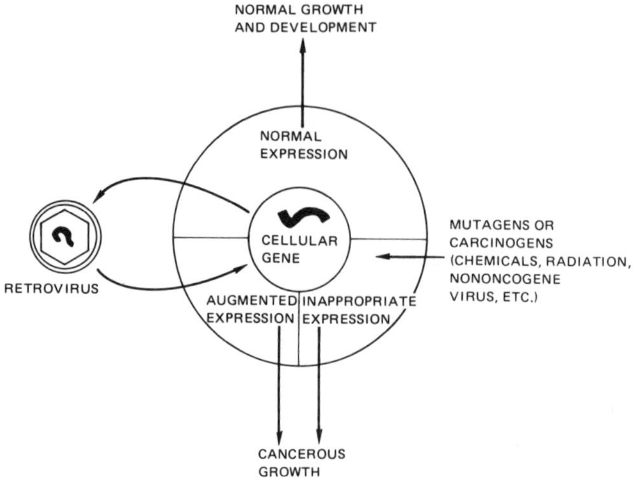

FIGURE 2–1 Cancer-gene concept. (*Source:* "Oncogenes," J. Michael Bishop, *Scientific American*, March 1982, © 1982 by Scientific American, Inc. All rights reserved.)

Cancer Proteins

The proteins encoded by oncogenes perform some specific biochemical activity within the cell, and it is that activity that turns a normal cell cancerous. The key to understanding malignancy, then, appears to lie within those proteins. Since oncogenes were first detected, a number of investigators have been trying to identify those proteins and determine where and how they act in the cell. Although most of the work to date has been performed on viral oncogenes, it provides insight into the biochemical activities of human oncogenes as well.

The first success came from the laboratory of Raymond L. Erickson at the University of Colorado School of Medicine. In 1977, he and Joan S. Brugge reported the isolation of the protein encoded by the *src* gene of the Rous sarcoma virus, the first retroviral oncogene detected. They named it pp60v-*src*. (The pp indicates that it is a phosphoprotein, the 60 refers to its molecular weight of 60,000 daltons, and the v-*src* indicates that its genetic origin is the viral *src* gene.)

Isolation proved to be the easy part: they and others are still trying to determine how the *src* protein induces cancerous growth. The first crucial step was to identify the protein by type. That was done by two groups, working independently: Erickson and his colleague Marc S. Collett, and Bishop, Varmus, and Arthur Levinson of the University of California School of Medicine in San Francisco. They found that the protein is a kinase, a type of enzyme that attaches phosphate ions to other proteins in a process known as protein phosphorylation. This discovery yielded one of the first clues to how the activity of a single protein could disrupt the normal behavior of a cell. Protein phosphorylation is thought to be one of the chief means by which the activities of growing cells are controlled. By phosphorylating cellular proteins, the *src* enzyme could conceivably change many aspects of cell structure and growth.

Soon after, it was found that the *src* protein works in an unconventional way. Most protein kinases attach proteins to one of two amino acids, threonine or serine. But Tony Hunter and Bartholomew M. Sefton of the Salk Institute for Biological Studies found that the *src* protein phosphorylates a different amino acid, tyrosine. Their finding spurred investigations to determine if tyrosine phosphorylation occurs in normal cells. Now it is clear that it does, and that it plays a role in the regulation of cell growth. This is just one of many instances in which the study of oncogenes is providing insight into the normal processes of cell growth and development.

As for the abnormal process, there is still only circumstantial evidence that protein phosphorylation is involved in the genesis of tumors. Hunter and other investigators are now locating and examining the targets of the *src* enzyme—the proteins it acts upon—to determine how their function is changed by phosphorylation. The *src* enzyme resides at the outskirts of the cell, bound to the plasma membrane. At least one of the proteins it attacks also resides in the membrane. Somehow this reaction at the cell's boundary influences events in the heart of the cell, the nucleus. Discovering how promises to be a lengthy process, for although one of the target proteins has been identified and dissected in fine detail, the investigators still know nothing of its normal function or how it is changed by phosphorylation.

A number of other oncogene proteins have also been characterized. Some, like the *src* enzyme, are protein kinases that phosphorylate tyrosine. Others are glycoproteins (proteins attached to carbohydrates) or nuclear proteins. Some work in the outer membrane, others in the cytoplasm or the nucleus. With one exception, the normal physiologic role of these genes is not known, nor is it understood how their activation can trigger cancerous growth. The exception is the protein encoded by the oncogene of a monkey retrovirus, v-*sis*, which bears an uncanny resemblance to the growth factor found in blood platelets. This lends support to the hypothesis that the benign proto-oncogenes are part of the cell's normal regulatory network, and that activated oncogenes may be distorted versions of regulatory genes.

Multistep Carcinogenesis

Perhaps the greatest uncertainty at present revolves around fitting what is known about the activation of an oncogene into the overall scheme of carcinogenesis. In human beings, tumorigenesis is known to be a complex process, arising from a number of discrete steps occurring within a cell. While the activation of an oncogene may be a necessary part of the process, it is not sufficient in and of itself to induce cancerous growth.

From the start, molecular biologists have suspected that several oncogenes may cooperate in transforming cells. That hunch has been borne out in recent experiments. Robert A. Weinberg of the Massachusetts Institute of Technology has found that some oncogenes are unable to transform cells in culture, yet when another oncogene is added, cancerous growth ensues. Perhaps tumors arise from the concerted action of a number of oncogenes, each representing one of the multiple steps in tumorigenesis. Investigators can only speculate on whether each oncogene must be activated separately, or if perhaps the activation of one oncogene triggers the next, and then the next, resulting in a cascade of reactions. Perhaps the proto-oncogenes are part of a delicately balanced regulatory network, and even a slight nudge is enough to tip the balance in favor of uncontrolled growth.

The study of oncogenes is providing the first glimpses into some of the genetic and biochemical changes that give rise to a cancer cell. It is too soon to predict exactly how this knowledge will be used to devise strategies to treat, cure, or prevent cancer. Investigators speculate that once the molecular events that start the disease are understood, it may be possible to interrupt them. It may, perhaps, be possible to develop biological agents specifically targeted to kill cancer cells, or to somehow disrupt the action of an oncogene protein. Such strategies, however, await the further understanding of the mechanisms by which oncogenes derange the cell, as well as the interactions among oncogenes and the external factors that trigger cancer.

3

Oncogenes in Human Cancer

In the early 1970s, after a decades-long search for the roots of cancer, molecular biologists at last identified a suspect: the oncogenes. By studying the retroviruses that cause cancer in animals, they had found a set of genes that acting alone or in concert could induce malignancy. Although these genes were first detected in viruses, it was soon learned that they were not bona fide viral genes at all. Instead, they are cellular genes that were picked up by the virus sometime during its evolution. These genes are found in benign form (in which case they are called proto-oncogenes) in the cells of higher animals, including human beings. Yet once they are captured by a virus and then reintroduced into an animal cell, they can trigger cancerous growth.

Since this discovery, one of the most intriguing questions in cancer research has been what, if anything, these oncogenes can

---

This chapter is based on the presentation given by Mariano Barbacid, National Cancer Institute-Frederick Cancer Research Facility, at the 1983 annual meeting of the Institute of Medicine.

reveal about human cancer. Do human cells also contain a set of genes that are responsible for the uncontrolled growth of tumor cells? If so, how are these putative human oncogenes activated? Probably not by viruses, or not often, because viruses may be only rarely involved in human cancer. Instead, most human cancers are thought to arise from exposure to certain chemicals or to physical carcinogens, such as the various forms of radiation. The obvious question is whether these agents somehow activate human oncogenes.

In the late 1970s, several groups of investigators began looking for oncogenes in human tumors. This was a separate endeavor from the work of other molecular biologists studying how retroviral oncogenes induce cancer. Instead, these researchers studied malignant human cells, using gene transfer and other techniques to try to determine the molecular basis of human cancer. Before long, however, the efforts of these distinct groups converged.

The Search for Human Oncogenes

Some of the first attempts to look for human oncogenes took place in the laboratories of Robert A. Weinberg at the Massachusetts Institute of Technology and Geoffrey M. Cooper of the Dana-Farber Cancer Institute at Harvard Medical School. In Weinberg's laboratory Chiaho Shih began looking for transforming genes in human and animal tumors. Using gene-transfer techniques, he isolated DNA from a variety of human tumor cell lines and introduced it into normal animal cells in culture. Those cells became cancerous. When the experiment was repeated using DNA from a normal human cell as a donor, there was no transformation. By transferring smaller and smaller pieces of DNA, the investigators were able to determine that the cancer-causing agent was a single gene, a human oncogene.

The next task was to isolate these human oncogenes and clone additional copies for study. Weinberg, Cooper, and scientists in two other laboratories, those of Mariano Barbacid at the National Cancer Institute and Michael Wigler of Cold Spring Harbor, began trying to fish out the oncogene activated in human bladder cancer. The work was far trickier than isolating a viral oncogene because the human cell contains tens of thousands of genes, as opposed to a handful in viruses.

Once the oncogene had been isolated, the four groups began scanning its nucleotide sequences, the procedure used to identify a gene. They were surprised to find that the gene was an old acquaintance: the human bladder oncogene was remarkably similar to an oncogene that had first been detected in the Harvey sarcoma virus, which causes tumors in rats. Similar results were obtained with oncogenes found in human lung and colon tumors: they turned out to be closely related to the oncogene of another rat tumor virus, the Kirsten strain of the sarcoma virus. In turn, both of those rat oncogenes—and thus the human oncogenes as well—are also related, belonging to a gene family known as *ras*.

With that discovery, the two groups of researchers—those investigating viral oncogenes and those looking for human oncogenes—realized that at least in some cases they were studying the same genes. The *ras* genes from the rat sarcoma viruses have innocuous counterparts in the rat genome from which they are derived. Similarly, investigators found that the human oncogenes also have related proto-oncogenes in normal cells. Moreover, it became immediately clear that these proto-oncogenes could be activated to a malignant state by two distinct routes—recombination with a virus or some nonviral mutation in a cell.

Several other human oncogenes have since been isolated. They are found in a broad range of human cancers: carcinomas of the bladder, breast, lung, and colon, as well as in fibrosarcomas, neuroblastomas, and leukemias. The same oncogene may be present in clinically unrelated cancers—there seems to be no correlation between a specific oncogene and a particular type of malignancy. Apparently, the nature of a tumor depends more on the type of tissue from which it derives than on which oncogene initiated the cancer process.

One puzzling finding is that these transforming genes have so far been detected in only 15 to 20 percent of human cancers, although these represent the broad range of human malignancies. There are two hypotheses. One is that oncogenes participate in all human cancers but that current assays are not sensitive enough to detect them. There is some evidence to support this, as the *myc* oncogene active in Burkitt lymphoma (discussed in Chapter 4) does not show up in some of these assays. The other possibility is that some human cancers arise by mechanisms that do not involve oncogenes.

Most of the human oncogenes belong to the *ras* family of genes. Three distinct *ras* genes, H-*ras*, K-*ras*, and N-*ras*, have been isolated to date. Although they differ structurally, they all code for the same or similar protein, known as p21, which has a molecular weight of 21,000 daltons. The normal role of these *ras* genes is not known, but as with the other oncogenes, they are thought to be involved in the regulation of cell growth and differentiation.

Most of the oncogenes detected to date in retroviruses and in mammalian cells also seem to fall into distinct groups or families. For molecular biologists, this is encouraging news. It suggests that the task of figuring out how these genes participate in cancer might not be as awesome as originally expected. Perhaps they code for a related group of proteins that perform a limited number of functions within the cell. The prevailing hypothesis is that the proto-oncogenes constitute part of a regulatory network, and when altered by a carcinogen they perform a slightly perverted version of this normal function.

A caveat is necessary when describing the transforming abilities of human oncogenes. They have been shown to transform only cells in culture, not cells in the living tissue of whole organisms. The use of the cell culture assay is a simplification—and not a foolproof one—of what is actually an extremely complex process. In the standard assay for transforming properties, genes are introduced into a line of cells, known as NIH 3T3, derived from connective tissue cells of a mouse. These cells are normal in most respects, except that they are immortal—that is, they have adapted to grow and divide indefinitely in a culture medium. There is abundant evidence suggesting that as the cells adapt to culture, they become more susceptible to transformation by oncogenes. Many biologists suspect that immortal cells are already well on their way to transformation, and that the introduction of an oncogene merely pushes them over the brink. Consequently, while this assay does detect malignant properties, it cannot be used as a definitive determination of the ability of a gene to transform cells *in vivo*.

Activation

The key question is how a cancer gene differs from a normal gene—what change endows it with transforming properties? In 1982, Weinberg at MIT, Barbacid at the National Cancer Institute, and Wigler at Cold Spring Harbor found the answer for the human bladder oncogene. In repeated tests, the investigators had been unable to detect a structural difference between this oncogene and its normal counterpart, the proto-oncogene. Nonetheless, the oncogene transformed cells in culture while the proto-oncogene did not. They realized that an extremely subtle change was involved—yet they never suspected just how subtle it would be. Working independently, all three groups found that the *ras* bladder oncogene differs from the normal gene in a single nucleotide substitution, the smallest genetic change possible.

A short review of molecular genetics may help to put this extraordinary finding in perspective. Nucleotides are the subunits of the double-stranded DNA molecule. Each of the two DNA strands is composed of a string of four nucleotide bases—adenine, guanine, cytosine, and thymine—arranged in varying order. The two strands are held together by weak bonds between the nucleotide bases: adenine on one strand always pairs with thymine on the other, as does guanine with cytosine.

A gene is a relatively short segment of DNA, composed of roughly 5,000 of these base pairs. Each gene contains the instructions for the synthesis of a specific protein. (Actually, protein synthesis is a two-step process—DNA is transcribed to a related molecule, RNA, then RNA is translated into protein.) The genetic code for a protein is contained in the sequence of nucleotide bases. A codon, or series of three nucleotides, such as TAT (thymine-adenine-thymine) codes for a specific amino acid, the basic component of a protein. During protein synthesis, the genetic code is "read" and amino acids are inserted into the growing protein chain according to the message of each codon.

The research teams of Barbacid, Weinberg, and Wigler found a single mutation in one of the 5,000 nucleotides of the active human bladder oncogene. In one spot in the gene, the normal codon GGC is replaced by GTC—a thymine has been substituted for a guanine. This tiny substitution, known as a point mutation, results in a change in the protein encoded by the gene. At one end of the oncogene's protein—specifically, at position 12—the amino

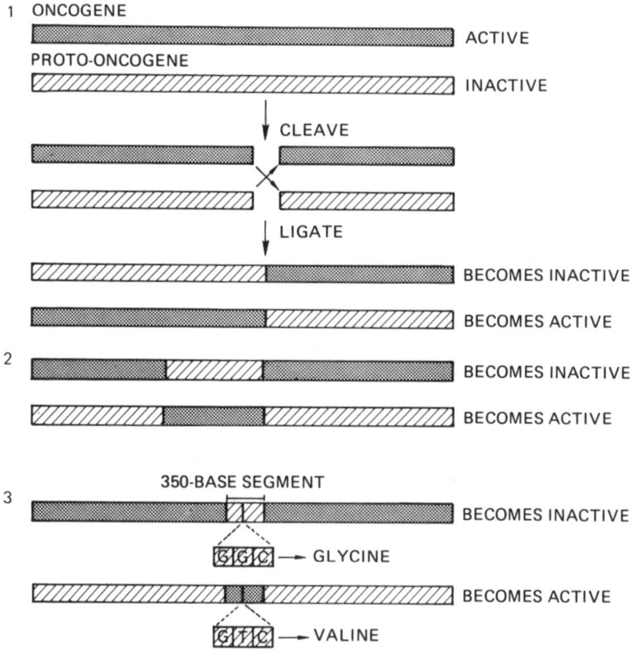

FIGURE 3–1 Point mutation in the *EJ* bladder carcinoma cell line. The proto-oncogene and the oncogene were cleaved at the same site and the resulting segments were joined. The resulting recombined genes were tested to see which had become active and which had lost activity. Successively smaller segments were similarly interchanged until a sequence only 350 bases in length was shown to be critical. This segment contains a single mutation: a guanine (G) in the proto-oncogene is converted to a thymine (T) in the oncogene, resulting in the specification of the amino acid valine rather than glycine. (SOURCE: "A Molecular Basis of Cancer," Robert A. Weinberg, *Scientific American*, November 1983, © 1983 by Scientific American, Inc. All rights reserved.)

acid valine is inserted instead of the usual glycine. Somehow, this substitution changes the protein such that it can trigger cancerous growth (see Figure 3-1).

The investigators had not expected to find a mutation in the protein-coding region of the gene. They had assumed instead that the regulatory region of the oncogene would be altered in some way. That seems to be the case in most of the retroviral oncogenes, at least. Researchers had already found that once those genes are put under viral control they are then turned on full blast. This excessive expression results in an overabundance of the protein product. In still other cases, investigators had found that oncogenes are present in multiple copies within a cell, also resulting in increased amounts of the protein. In both instances, too much of an otherwise normal protein seems to contribute to the malignant growth. For the human bladder oncogene, however, the change appears to be qualitative, not quantitative. The oncogene seems to be expressed in the correct amount, but in a slightly different form. Thus, an altered rather than overabundant protein seems to be at fault.

It is not known what causes this mutation in the oncogene, or how the altered protein might act to induce cancer. Through computer analysis, investigators have recently found that the substitution of valine for glycine dramatically changes the structure of the protein. Presumably, this change in turn alters the protein's interactions with other molecules in the cell. Efforts are now under way to determine the biochemical activities of both the normal and transforming protein.

Cause or Consequence?

Although it is tempting to suppose that the altered oncogene initiates the tumor, it could nonetheless be a consequence, not a cause. The point mutation in the human bladder oncogene could be a product of the genetic disarray of a cancer cell. The case for the altered gene as cause has been strengthened, however, by a finding reported by Barbacid and his colleagues in early 1984. The NCI researchers, Barbacid, Eugenio Santos, Dionisio Martin-Zanca, and E. Premkumar Reddy, were aided by Marco A. Pierotti and

Guiseppe Della Porta of the National Institute for the Study and Cure of Tumors in Milan, Italy. In cells of a squamous lung tumor removed from a 66-year-old man, the investigators found the active, mutated oncogene. Yet in normal bronchial tissue from the same patient, the mutation was not present. Thus, the mutated oncogene is not a part of the patient's normal genetic complement. Rather, it is clearly associated with the development of a cancer. As Barbacid says, it is hard to think that it is not responsible for that cancer. Perhaps, the researchers speculate, the gene was mutated by a chemical in cigarette smoke, for the patient was a heavy smoker.

Barbacid and his colleagues then turned to animals to study the chemical initiation of cancer. They hoped to discern the method of attack of a chemical carcinogen—specifically, whether it activated an oncogene. They induced breast cancer in female rats by injecting them with nitroso-methylurea, a potent chemical carcinogen. These induced tumors were found to contain transforming genes, while the breast cells from untreated rats did not.

Again, the transforming gene turned out to be the now-familiar *ras* gene, activated by the same point mutation that occurs in human tumors. Of all the possible changes in the gene's 5,000 base pairs, the switch occurred in exactly the same one in all of the treated animals.

Although more work must be done, this is the clearest indication yet to Barbacid and his colleagues that the chemical carcinogen, acting either directly or indirectly, mutates the proto-oncogene, and that such a mutation is responsible for the development of the tumor. Barbacid emphasizes that what is seen in the laboratory is just a small piece of the process of carcinogenesis—that the activation of a single oncogene probably accounts for one of numerous biochemical changes necessary for a tumor to develop. That one change, however, appears to be critical, Barbacid says. By using induced tumors in rats to study chemical carcinogenesis, the NCI researchers hope to learn the exact role of oncogenes in human cancer. So far, their work has provided another piece of evidence, albeit indirect, that some human cancers arise when a chemical or other environmental insult activates an oncogene, creating a slightly altered protein, which then disrupts normal cell behavior.

To date, the point mutation has been found only in the *ras* gene. Another human oncogene, the *myc* gene, has recently been shown to be switched on by a different mechanism, chromosome rearrangement. Additional mechanisms of activation probably remain to be discovered. In short, there seem to be many ways to convert a normal gene to a cancer gene.

4

Broken Chromosomes

When biologists first peered inside tumor cells, they found that many of the chromosomes, the rodlike structures that carry the genes, were strikingly abnormal. Many chromosomes had been broken apart; sometimes segments of DNA appeared in extra copies. Sometimes pieces were either missing entirely or else had been flipped over or shuffled among chromosomes.

In the past few years, geneticists have developed various techniques to keep track of the movements of chromosomes. Jorge Yunis of the University of Minnesota, for instance, stains tiny bands of chromosomes, often containing as few as 10 genes (an entire chromosome typically contains 1,000 genes). He can then follow that band should it break off of one chromosome and hook up with another or change position on its own chromosome.

Using this technique, Yunis examined the malignant cells in

This chapter is based on the presentation given by Philip Leder, Harvard University School of Medicine, at the 1983 annual meeting of the Institute of Medicine.

tumors of 380 patients with various forms of cancer. Ninety-five percent of the cases showed some kind of chromosome defect—such as a translocation or a deletion. In 72 percent of the cases, the defect was specific to the type of cancer with which it was associated.

Geneticists have long suspected that these chromosomal abnormalities are somehow involved in the genesis of tumors. Yet until recently, they had no idea how.

An answer is emerging in large part from another line of cancer research. As geneticists were cataloging the chromosome defects in cancer cells, molecular biologists were pursuing specific cancer-causing genes, the oncogenes. Part of the normal genetic complement of all cells, these oncogenes can be stirred to malignant action when they are disturbed in some way, perhaps by the action of a mutagen or a virus. There is now evidence that chromosome rearrangement may be one means by which an oncogene is activated. In other words, cancer may arise when an oncogene on one chromosome is moved to a new position on another chromosome.

Burkitt Lymphoma

The evidence about chromosome rearrangement comes largely from the study of Burkitt lymphoma, a cancer that primarily afflicts children in Central Africa and New Guinea, and a related cancer that occurs in mice. Both this mouse plasmacytoma and Burkitt lymphoma are malignancies of the B-cells, a type of cell in the immune system that produces antibodies—the forces the body musters to ward off viruses and other foreign invaders. The B-cells of Burkitt victims show a specific chromosomal abnormality known as a translocation. In roughly 80 percent of the cases, a piece of chromosome 8 changes places with a piece of chromosome 14. In the remainder, the translocation occurs between chromosome 8 and chromosome 2 or chromosome 8 and chromosome 22. A similar translocation occurs in mouse plasmacytoma. (The chromosomes are numbered according to size; in human beings, the largest is chromosome 1, the smallest is chromosome 22. The sex chromosomes are known as X and Y.)

The first hint that these translocations might induce malignancy came not from cancer research but from basic investigations into the genetics of the immune system. One of the most perplexing aspects of the immune system is its incredible diversity—how is the body able to produce millions of different antibodies to the substances it encounters? Each antibody protein is encoded by a specific gene, so the answer must lie there. Several researchers, including Philip Leder of Harvard University and Leroy Hood of the California Institute of Technology, have been studying these genes, which are located at particular sites known as the immunoglobulin loci, on various chromosomes.

The details have been worked out in the past few years. It turns out that the genes for specific antibodies are made when tiny bits of DNA—smaller than a gene—from a number of chromosomes join together. In a developing B-cell, chromosomes constantly break and then rejoin as bits of DNA are shuffled into new arrangements, each coding for a distinct protein, an antibody. These genes are then actively transcribed, that is, they are switched on and then direct synthesis of the antibody protein.

At the sites of the antibody genes, then, chromosome rearrangement is the norm. It was not long before several researchers noted the similarity between these normal events and the aberrant translocations that occur—with devastating effect—in Burkitt lymphoma. Suspicion that the normal process might somehow be involved in carcinogenesis increased when various investigators began mapping the antibody genes to their respective chromosomes. They found that the antibody genes reside on three chromosomes, numbers 14, 2, and 22—precisely the same chromosomes that exchange pieces with chromosome 8 in Burkitt lymphoma.

The connection was not lost on George Klein, who was studying mouse plasmacytoma at the Karolinska Institute in Sweden. He proposed that chromosome 8 must harbor a proto-oncogene—a benign gene that has malignant potential. Burkitt lymphoma would arise, he reasoned, when that oncogene was moved from chromosome 8 into the antibody-producing region on chromosome 14, where it would be switched on and expressed along with the antibody genes.

Following Klein's hunch, several other laboratories began looking for a proto-oncogene on chromosome 8. Some of the key researchers in this effort include Leder, Hood, Carlo Croce at the Wistar Institute, Ricardo Dalla-Favera and Robert Gallo of the National Cancer Institute, Michael Cole of the St. Louis University School of Medicine, and Kenneth Marcu of the State University of New York at Stonybrook.

The cellular *myc* gene, originally isolated from a chicken retrovirus, seemed a likely candidate for the suspected oncogene, as William S. Hayward of the Memorial Sloan-Kettering Cancer Center had found that this gene is activated in other forms of lymphoma. Hayward, Gallo, and Croce found that indeed, the *myc* gene is located on chromosome 8, on the segment that is swapped in Burkitt lymphoma. At the same time, Leder and his colleagues found exactly where on chromosome 14 the *myc* gene is inserted—into or very close to the site of an active antibody gene (see Figure 4-1). They have subsequently found that the oncogene is also

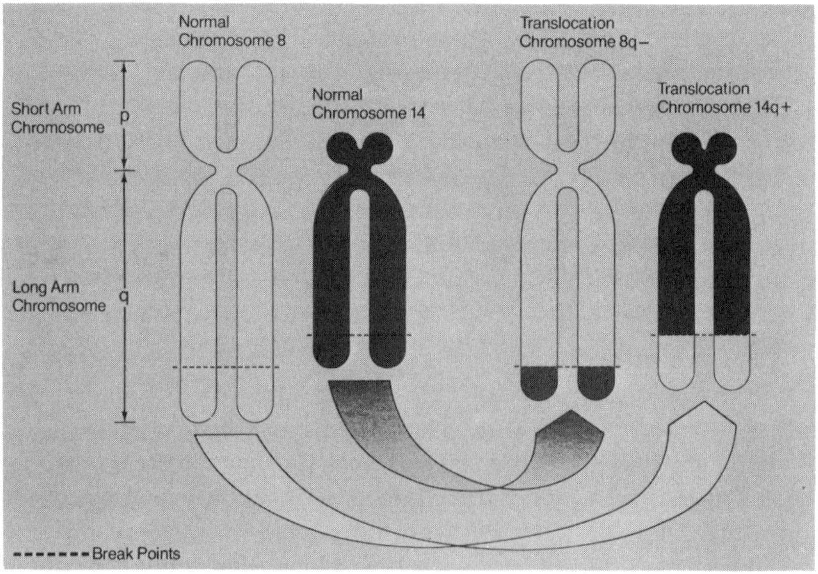

FIGURE 4–1 Chromosome translocation in Burkitt lymphoma. (SOURCE: Bristol-Myers Company/University of Chicago Cancer Research Center.)

inserted into the antibody gene sites on chromosomes 2 and 22. Other researchers, including Marcu, Croce, and Hood, found that in mouse plasmacytoma the *myc* gene was also translocated into the region of the antibody gene.

Uncertain Data

In its new position, the once-benign *myc* gene appears to be suddenly malignant. Yet the exact way in which the translocation activates the oncogene remains obscure. Similarly, there are few clues to how the activated oncogene might cause Burkitt lymphoma.

There are two possibilities. The translocation could disturb the regulation of the gene, turning it on at the wrong time or in the wrong amount, as has been found for many retroviral oncogenes. Alternately, the reshuffling could mutate the coding region of the gene, resulting in the production of a slightly different protein. Another human oncogene, the *ras* gene, has recently been found to be switched on in that way.

Some evidence exists to support each theory. Several investigators have found that in Burkitt cells the translocated *myc* gene is overexpressed—it is turned on too high and is making too much of its protein product. This finding fits in well with Klein's original hypothesis. He had postulated that when the gene was inserted into the antibody site it would fall under different control signals and be overexpressed. The excess protein would then spur malignant growth. This theory is buttressed by the finding that levels of *myc* expression are elevated in other, non-Burkitt tumors.

Other research points to an altered protein caused by mutation or other damage to the gene. At St. Louis University, for instance, Michael Cole has evidence that a segment of the *myc* gene may be lost in the translocation.

Sorting out these apparently conflicting data will take some time. Investigators are just beginning to characterize the normal *myc* gene—a crucial step in determining the difference between the normal gene and the transforming one. Comparisons of the level of expression of the two versions of the gene are speculative, as little is known about its expression in normal cells. Similarly, not much is known about either the physical properties of the normal *myc* protein or its function within the cell.

Once these and other results are in, it may turn out that the two theories—a regulatory disturbance or an altered gene product—are both correct. In Burkitt cells, the translocations do not always occur in exactly the same place; several distinct crossover points between chromosomes 8 and 14 have been found. In some cases, the *myc* gene is not inserted into the antibody gene site at all, although it is translocated to a nearby site on the same chromosome. Perhaps the *myc* gene can be activated in a number of ways depending on where the break occurs.

A Regulatory Disturbance

The newest evidence suggests that a regulatory disturbance is the major culprit in Burkitt lymphoma. Much of this evidence has come from Philip Leder and his colleagues at Harvard University, Jim Battey, Christopher Moulding, William Murphy, Huntington Potter, Timothy Stewart, and Rebecca Taub, and Gilbert Lenoir of the World Health Organization's International Agency for Research on Cancer.

They have found that the structure of the coding region of the translocated *myc* gene is identical to its normal, unrearranged counterpart. This strongly suggests that their protein products must also be identical. If so, then the transforming gene and the normal gene must differ chiefly in their expression, at least in the particular line of Burkitt cells that the Harvard team examined.

The geneticists had expected to find overexpression of the translocated *myc* gene in Burkitt cells. Yet their measurements revealed that expression of the translocated oncogene was only slightly, if at all, higher than that of a *myc* gene in a noncancerous B-cell in culture. Other investigators have consistently found a slight elevation in expression of the translocated *myc* gene. In yet other cases, a sizable, 20- to 40-fold increase in expression has been detected In short, although the gene appears to be aberrantly expressed in most cases, the level of expression varies dramatically.

Investigators have been perplexed by the inconsistent findings. Given this wide variation, Leder began to think it unlikely that the elevated expression of the *myc* gene was at fault in Burkitt lymphoma, or not so simply. In particular, he wondered why such a minimal increase in expression should confer transforming properties on a gene. He began to suspect that a more complex regulatory disturbance had occurred.

In some instances, Leder's group has been able to study a normal and a rearranged *myc* gene within the same cell. (Genes are always present in two copies, known as alleles—one on the maternal chromosome and one on the paternal. In most Burkitt cells, only one of the chromosomes has been rearranged, the other is unchanged.) In comparing expression of the two versions of the *myc* gene, the Harvard researchers have detected subtle changes in expression, specifically, in the way in which the gene is transcribed. They have also noted another intriguing phenomenon: in Burkitt cells, the translocated gene is active—that is, it is producing protein—while the normal gene is silent.

Leder and his colleagues have now found that although the protein-coding region of the translocated *myc* gene is intact, another part of the gene has been damaged by the translocation. They think that these mutations occur in the region of the gene that regulates its expression. Usually the damage is slight, a small alteration in the nucleotide sequences. But sometimes this entire control region is missing.

Kathleen Kelly, another researcher in Leder's laboratory, has been examining expression of the *myc* gene in normal cells. The *myc* gene is thought to be involved in cell growth and division, perhaps in mitosis, or DNA replication, or transcription. In collaboration with Brent Cochran and Charles Stiles of the Dana-Farber Cancer Center, Kelly is trying to determine at what stage in the cell cycle the gene is normally active. They have found that expression of the *myc* gene appears tightly controlled: it is switched on at a very specific time, as the cell is moving from the resting phase (through which a cell must pass in order to divide) to the growth phase. The rest of the time it is silent, presumably blocked by some kind of repressive control.

Leder suspects that during translocation, the *myc* gene slips loose of the repressive controls. Then, because the control region of the translocated gene is damaged or missing, whatever usually shuts off the gene can no longer affect it at its new site. This would explain why the translocated gene is active in a Burkitt cell and the normal allele is usually silent. The important consequence of this deregulation, Leder postulates, is not overproduction of a protein, although that may be involved, but rather a change in the *time* the gene is expressed. Because *myc* expression is tightly related to the cycle of cell division and growth, a change in its timing would disrupt the cycle's normal pattern.

The action of the *myc* gene alone is not sufficient to induce Burkitt lymphoma. Leder and others suspect that the gene collaborates with other, as yet unknown oncogenes to transform the cell. Several activated oncogenes have been detected in many other tumors. Robert A. Weinberg of MIT recently found evidence of actual oncogene collaboration. He has shown that in some non-Burkitt cell line systems, the *myc* gene is unable to transform cells alone; it requires the action of another oncogene. Indeed, since the *myc* gene was detected, another transforming gene, known as *Blym*, has recently turned up in Burkitt cells. Whether it collaborates with the *myc* gene, and if so in what way, remains to be determined.

Spontaneous Carcinogenesis

Details remain to be worked out on exactly how the translocation activates the *myc* gene. Yet even at this preliminary stage, the research in Burkitt cells provides a model for spontaneous carcinogenesis, or cancer that arises apparently without the action of a virus or a mutagen.

In the past decade or so, biologists have become increasingly aware that genes are not permanently fixed in one place. They can change position on their chromosome and are sometimes shuffled between different chromosomes. The translocations in Burkitt cells suggest that some cancers arise when this normal process goes awry—when genes end up in the wrong place. It is intriguing to view Burkitt lymphoma as a perversion of the normal process of antibody production. In a normal B-cell, chromosome 14 exchanges pieces with chromosomes 2 and 22. In Burkitt cells, the instructions seem to have been muddled, and instead, these three chromosomes begin exhanging bits with chromosome 8, which bears the *myc* oncogene.

Chromosomal abnormalities are not restricted to Burkitt cells; as mentioned earlier, some type of chromosome defect occurs in most cancer cells. Cells isolated from many types of leukemias also show chromosomal translocations, and investigators have recently detected oncogenes on the chromosomes involved in these switches. In other types of cancer, such as solid tumors, the most frequent abnormality is a deletion of part of a chromosome. Research is under way to determine if these other chromosomal defects also affect an oncogene.

5

The Epidemiology of Diet and Cancer

The causes of cancer are extraordinarily difficult to discern. A small number of cancers are clearly of familial, or genetic, origin. Yet the majority seem to be caused either by spontaneous metabolic events or by specific external factors—substances encountered in the course of normal living.

Many of the clues to the origins of cancer have come from epidemiologists, who search for the causes of disease among the broad characteristics of a population. Like detectives, epidemiologists work backwards from the crime: they study the incidence and distribution of a disease and then try to deduce the factors that caused it. They look for any telltale differences among people—such as their race or age, the foods they eat, or their exposure to viruses or industrial pollutants—that might explain why some are afflicted with a disease and others are spared.

This chapter is based on the presentation given by Anthony B. Miller, National Cancer Institute of Canada, University of Toronto, at the 1983 annual meeting of the Institute of Medicine.

As such, epidemiology is descriptive and suggestive. It uncovers associations, points to populations at risk, provides clues about factors to blame, and raises hypotheses for further study.

Over the past few decades, epidemiologists have been able to map the global patterns of cancer occurrence. They have found striking variations in both the incidence and types of cancers that occur in different countries, which suggests that external factors, including lifestyle, may be responsible. These variations are not due to ethnic origin, for when people migrate from one country to another, they tend to acquire the pattern of cancer typical of their new home.

Epidemiologists now believe that 80 to 90 percent of all cancers are caused by external, or environmental, factors. Identifying the culprits will be an arduous task, for the long list of suspects includes smoking, diet, industrial chemicals, substances in air and water, the regions where a person lives or works, viruses and other infectious agents, and other personal habits. Nonetheless, many scientists see the role of external factors as the most encouraging finding to emerge from cancer research: it means that cancer may be largely preventable.

The Search Narrows

Some of the environmental causes of cancer are fairly obvious. As early as the eighteenth century, occupational exposure to certain toxic chemicals was implicated by epidemiological studies when an English surgeon, Percival Pott, noted the abnormally high incidence of scrotal cancer among chimney sweeps. Later epidemiological studies revealed that workers who handled aniline dye faced an increased risk of bladder cancer. More recently, the incidence of lung cancer in coastal regions of the United States has been linked to exposure to asbestos in the shipbuilding industry during World War II.

About 30 years ago, epidemiologists noticed an association between cigarette smoking and lung cancer. Many years elapsed before their suspicions were borne out in laboratory experiments, but now tobacco is thought to account for one-third of all cancer deaths in the United States alone. Lung cancer is the most prevalent form of cancer in the Western nations, and its incidence has been rising throughout this century as an increasing number of men, and later women, started smoking. Cigarette smoking also contributes to cancers at other sites, including the bladder and probably the pancreas and kidney.

Recently, suspicion has turned to both the intended and unintended products of industrialization, such as industrial chemicals or pollution from oil and gas consumption. So far, the fear that the environment has become increasingly carcinogenic has not been confirmed by epidemiological studies. Although the number of people who develop and die of cancer has risen, much of the increase is related to smoking. The rest can be largely explained by increasing life expectancy: more people are living to the age when cancer usually takes its toll. When adjusted for age, the incidence of those cancers unrelated to smoking has actually declined since World War II. Nevertheless, industrial products are constantly changing; new chemicals are being synthesized. It is not known whether these new products will increase the cancer risk.

Meanwhile, it is clear that a major cause of today's cancers remains to be discovered. Given the fairly constant cancer rate of the past 30 years, it would seem that some longstanding aspects of lifestyle, such as diet, are responsible. Diet—the foods and portions people eat and the method of preparation—varies greatly from society to society and could account for many of the observed differences in international cancer incidence. But it has been only in the past two decades that cancer researchers have begun to suspect that certain features of an abundant, apparently normal diet could be related to cancer.

An Imprecise Tool

Of all the possible external causes of cancer, diet is perhaps the most difficult to evaluate. It is far easier to determine whether and how much people smoke than to find out what and how much they eat, or particularly what they ate a decade or two ago. The problem is not simply the vagaries of memory or the variation in individual eating habits, but a general paucity of knowledge about the contemporary food supply. Foods are complex substances, the exact composition of which is often not known. The increasing reliance on processed foods compounds the difficulty.

To determine dietary intake, epidemiologists often rely on indirect data, some of which have been collected for entirely different purposes. One measure is national per capita food intake data, also known as food disappearance data, which takes into account the amount of food produced in a country as well as the amount exported, imported, fed to livestock, lost in storage, etc. Another approach is the household food inventory, in which individuals record purchases or menus.

Using these techniques, epidemiologists have in the past two decades uncovered specific associations between types of cancer and various diets. They have documented a correlation between the diet of affluent societies, for instance, and cancers of certain organs—primarily breast, colon, and uterus. They have identified some foods that seem to increase the risk of cancer and others that seem to decrease it. These studies, however, reveal only associations; in none of them has diet been proved to cause cancer.

Nonetheless, when numerous epidemiological studies repeatedly turn up the same associations, the weight of evidence becomes difficult to ignore. That is what happened with smoking and cancer some 20 years ago. And that is what is happening now with diet and cancer. In addition, laboratory studies have tended to support the epidemiological data. The evidence is now strong enough for a number of leading scientists, including a recent committee of the National Research Council (NRC),[1] to conclude that diet is associated with many common cancers. (At this preliminary stage, however, the NRC committee could not determine exactly how much cancer can be attributed to diet.) A more difficult task will be to determine precisely which dietary components are either protective or to blame and the mechanisms by which they influence the development of cancer.

---

[1] The Committee on Diet, Nutrition, and Cancer of the National Research Council. The studies described in this chapter are discussed in greater detail in its report, *Diet, Nutrition, and Cancer*. Washington, D.C.: National Academy Press, 1982.

Migrant Studies

Some of the first evidence that diet might be related to cancer came from studies of migrants. In the 1960s and 1970s, a number of epidemiologists determined the cancer incidence among certain populations that had migrated from one country to another. A consistent pattern emerged: for first-generation migrants, the pattern of certain cancers remained similar to that in the country of origin, or perhaps intermediate between the old and new country. Yet after one or more generations, migrants acquired the cancers characteristic of the host country.

For example, among the Japanese who migrated to the western United States in the early 1900s, the first generation was found to have a far lower mortality rate for breast cancer than the Caucasian population. (In the United States and other affluent nations, breast and colon and rectal, or colorectal, cancer are particularly prevalent.) By the second generation, the mortality from breast cancer had increased dramatically, and by the third generation was almost identical to that of the native population. This occurred without any outbreeding in the Japanese community—instead, it was due to acculturation.

Similar changes have been observed among migrants to Israel, who come both from affluent and less developed nations. The Israel Cancer Registry provides a wealth of information for epidemiologists, for it regularly publishes data on the incidence of cancer according to the birthplace of its citizens. First-generation migrants show a marked increase in colorectal cancer: one study showed that for middle-aged women who had migrated from Asia and Africa, the incidence of colorectal cancer increased by 39 percent over a 10-year period. For women born in Israel, the incidence increased by 102 percent during that same period. Other migrants to Israel who came from Western European countries, the United States, and Canada—where colorectal cancer is much more prevalent—showed very little increase. A similar pattern occurs for breast cancer—Asian and African migrants and those born in Israel show a marked increase, while the incidence for migrants from Western nations remains stable. Thus, the biggest changes in colorectal and breast cancer incidence seem to be among migrants

TABLE 5–1 Comparison of Rates of Colorectal Cancer Among Native and Migrant Jewish Females Ages 35–64, in Israel

Native Country	Increase in Incidence (percent)			
	1960–1966	1967–1971	1972–1976	1966–1976
Israel	17.0	26.6	34.3	102
Africa/Asia	11.9	13.9	16.5	39
Europe/N. America	35.2	35.7	39.4	12

(*Source:* Anthony B. Miller, National Cancer Institute of Canada.)

TABLE 5–2 Comparison of Rates of Breast Cancer Among Native and Migrant Jewish Females Ages 35–64, in Israel

Native Country	Increase in Incidence (percent)			
	1960–1966	1967–1971	1972–1976	1966–1976
Israel	85.9	125.2	132.3	54
Africa/Asia	54.0	60.5	133.6	49
Europe/N. America	132.4	133.6	136.2	3

(*Source:* Anthony B. Miller, National Cancer Institute of Canada.)

from Asia and Africa who are adopting Israel's more affluent life-style (see Tables 5-1 and 5-2).

What is particularly interesting is that the change in the incidence of breast cancer occurs rapidly—the incidence is as high for the foreign-born migrants from Asia and Africa as it is for natives of Israel. This is in direct contrast to the pattern observed in Japanese migrants. In that group, the incidence of colon cancer increased rapidly, while the changes in rates of breast cancer did not occur for one or often two generations. Epidemiologists suspect that this may reflect different rates of acculturation. Some migrant groups retain many of their cultural habits, including diet, for several generations. This has been shown for some Japanese populations in Canada, who after 35 to 50 years in their new country continued to eat more fish and rice and less beef, potatoes, bread, and milk than the Canadian-born population.

Religious Groups

Certain religious groups have proved to be incredibly fruitful subjects for epidemiologists, as they follow distinct diets that differ from that of the population at large. Most of these studies of the association between diet and cancer have focused on cancers of the gastrointestinal tract and the breast and other tissues subject to hormonal influence, as nutrition is known to affect hormone levels.

The Seventh Day Adventists abstain from tobacco and alcohol, and roughly half of them are lacto-ovovegetarians—that is, they eat dairy products but no meat. In several studies, Roland Phillips and his colleagues at Loma Linda University in California have found that this diet seems to protect against colorectal cancer: Seventh Day Adventists had lower rates of both this diet-related cancer and smoking-related cancers than did a control group of comparable age, sex, and social status. The incidence of breast cancer was also reduced, but not significantly.

The Mormons abstain from alcohol, tobacco, coffee, and tea. Many follow a diet rich in grains, fruits, and vegetables, with a moderate consumption of meat. The incidence of colorectal cancer is also lower among Mormons, according to a study by Joseph L. Lyons of the University of Utah in Salt Lake City.

In India, the incidence of cancer varies dramatically among different religious groups. The Parsis, who eat a Western-style diet, have a much higher incidence of breast, colon, and rectal cancer than do the Hindus, who generally follow a strict vegetarian diet.

Which Dietary Components?

These broad, descriptive surveys point to several dietary components, such as fat and animal protein, that might influence cancer. Other studies have examined the association between specific dietary components and other variables with cancer incidence and mortality.

In 1975, Bruce Armstrong and Sir Richard Doll of Oxford University reported the results of their massive study, which included over 30 nations and correlated the incidence and mortality rates of cancer at nearly 30 sites or organs with a range of dietary and other variables. The strongest correlations were for meat and fat intake with cancers of the colorectum, breast, uterus, and ovary. They also found associations between total fat intake and testicular and kidney cancer.

Armstrong and Doll also detected other direct correlations: intestinal cancer with sugar; pancreatic cancer with eggs, animal protein, and fat; ovary and bladder cancer with fats and oils. Some inverse relationships also came to light: gastric cancer with meat, animal protein, and fat; cervical cancer with protein and fruit.

Kenneth Carroll of the University of Western Ontario calculated that there was a strong correlation worldwide between per capita total fat intake and age-adjusted mortality from breast cancer. The highest mortality rates are found in those nations with the highest fat intake—the United States, the United Kingdom, and Canada. The lowest rate is found in Japan and other Eastern countries, where people consume far less fat. The correlation was strongest for total fat, almost as strong for animal fat, but nearly absent for vegetable fat.

In Armstrong and Doll's study, many of the dietary variables, especially animal protein and animal fat, were correlated with each other and with gross national product. Other studies have also revealed a correlation between particular cancers and socioeconomic status, which is a major indicator of diet and lifestyle. In the United States, breast cancer—the leading cancer among women—is correlated with higher socioeconomic status among postmenopausal women. Cancer of the colon and rectum in men is also linked with higher socioeconomic status. For both sexes, renal cancer is more prevalent at higher socioeconomic levels. By contrast, stomach and lip cancer appear to be predominately found among less affluent groups. Similar findings have been observed in other countries. When the data are adjusted for occupation, strong correlations still remain, suggesting that social class is a major indicator of cancer risk.

Other variables, which may in fact be nutrition-related, have also been found to be associated along with diet in the incidence of or mortality from cancer. Gregory Gray and his colleagues at the University of California at Los Angeles found that in addition to intake of animal protein and fat, a woman's height and weight are positively associated with breast cancer. Other studies have shown that the risk of dying of breast cancer increases proportionately with body weight.

Epidemiologists can begin to move from the detection of associations to inferences about causality when they collect data from individuals rather than rely on broad estimates of a population's diet. By interviewing individuals, epidemiologists can get a far more accurate assessment of actual dietary intake, although the technique is not foolproof. For one, epidemiologists must trust in an individual's recall and accuracy. In addition, the underlying assumption is that the current diet reflects the individual's diet at the time the cancer was initiated, one or perhaps two decades ago.

One approach is the case-control study, in which investigators collect detailed information on dietary intake from individuals who have a particular type of cancer. This is then compared with dietary intake of a selected control population whose members do not have cancer. This difficult and time-consuming procedure has been used most frequently to study breast and colorectal cancer, examining in greater detail the associations brought to light by the descriptive and correlation studies.

Breast Cancer

A major study on breast cancer was completed in Canada in 1978 by Anthony B. Miller of the National Cancer Institute of Canada and the University of Toronto. He and his colleagues collected dietary intake data on six nutrients from 400 breast cancer cases and 400 controls. For both pre- and postmenopausal women, the strongest correlation was with total fat consumption. For premenopausal women, there were also weaker associations with saturated fat and cholesterol. Of major importance in these investigations is evidence for dose-response—does the risk increase proportionately with dose? For total fat, Miller's group initially found no evidence of a dose-response ratio, but their subsequent, more detailed analyses suggest that for saturated fat, the risk may be greater with increasing consumption.

Miller and his colleagues have estimated that a larger share of breast cancer can be attributed to high fat intake than it can to the other variables known to be involved in the etiology of the disease, such as age at first pregnancy, family history of breast cancer, and weight.

Another study reveals a similar correlation. Jay Lubin and his colleagues at the National Cancer Institute and the Cross Cancer Institute in Edmonton, Alberta, have found that risk of breast cancer increases significantly with frequent consumption of beef and other red meat, pork, and desserts—all of which reflect fat consumption.

Colorectal Cancer

A greater number of case-control studies have explored the relation of diet and colorectal cancer. Diverse subgroups have been examined—blacks in California, Japanese in Hawaii, and other groups in the Caribbean countries, Scandinavia, Norway, Australia, New York, and Canada. Some of the results have been conflicting—perhaps reflecting differences in accuracy of the various methodologies—but in all, they point to a strong association between total fat intake and colorectal cancer. The association appears to be particularly strong for saturated fat.

Several early, descriptive studies have turned up what seems to be a protective role for dietary fiber from grains and vegetables. As mentioned earlier, the Seventh Day Adventists have a low incidence of colon cancer. Similarly, the Punjabis of northern India, who eat a diet rich in cellulose, roughage, and vegetable fiber, have almost no colon cancer. Yet efforts to document these associations in case-control studies have yielded inconsistent results.

In several of these studies, epidemiologists have found that victims of colon cancer do consume less fiber than do controls. But one difficulty with these studies is that the amount of fiber in the diet is usually not measured; instead, it is estimated from the intake of certain vegetables, fruits, and whole grains. In one study that did quantify fiber intake, the investigators did not find a protective effect for fiber. They did observe, however, that incidence of colon cancer was inversely related to intake of one fiber component, the pentosan fraction, which is found in whole wheat products and other foods. That may help to explain the different results of these case-control studies: it might not be fiber per se but rather a particular component or components that protect against colon cancer.

People who eat a lot of vegetables also tend to fare better in terms of colon and rectal cancer. A number of studies suggest a protective role for cruciferous vegetables—cabbage, broccoli, cauliflower, and brussels sprouts. For instance, Saxon Graham of the State University of New York at Buffalo found that individuals who rarely eat these vegetables—once a month or less frequently—face the highest risk of colon cancer. The lowest risk was for those who consume cruciferous vegetables weekly. He also found a protective effect against rectal cancer, though it was far weaker. Anthony Miller and others have also documented a weak protective effect for these vegetables. At this stage, it is still unclear which component of the vegetables is responsible.

Accumulating Evidence

Epidemiological studies are only one-half of the evidence implicating diet in the development or prevention of cancer. Laboratory studies are now under way to test the various hypotheses. The results to date have tended to confirm the epidemiological data. For instance, a number of nutritive and non-nutritive compounds present in cruciferous vegetables have been shown to inhibit carcinogenesis in cells in culture. Yet even in laboratory experiments, it is still not clear which components exert this beneficial effect.

Similarly, experiments on animals have consistently shown that dietary fats promote tumorigenesis (the formation of tumors), especially in the breast and colon. When fat intake is increased from 10 to 40 percent of total calories in the diet of laboratory animals, tumor incidence in various tissues also rises.

On the positive side, the consumption of some ingredients in high-fiber foods, such as cellulose and bran, has been shown to inhibit the induction of colon cancer by certain chemical carcinogens, but not consistently.

Although laboratory studies support the epidemiological findings, it is still too soon to say with certainty whether the specific associations between dietary components and different cancers are causal. More basic research is necessary to determine the mechanisms by which diet might trigger the development of cancer.

Some clues about possible mechanisms have come from studying animals in which tumors have been induced by known chemical carcinogens. In most cases, carcinogenesis seems to be a multistep process. It begins when the animal is exposed to an initiating agent, presumably a mutagen that damages DNA. Often initiation does not appear to be sufficient to give rise to a tumor; the action of other agents, known as promoters, is necessary to complete the process. Promoters may not be mutagens; instead, they seem to modify or accelerate the normal processes of cell differentiation and promote cell proliferation.

Dietary components could influence either the early or late stages of carcinogenesis—both stages are poorly understood. Many carcinogenic initiators seem to be created by metabolic interactions within the cell—that is, one chemical is converted to another, carcinogenic form within the cell. Some dietary components may actually be initiating substances; others may modify different substances within the cell, converting them to initiators.

Even less is known about the late stages of carcinogenesis, although preliminary evidence suggests that diet may exert its greatest influence there. Some dietary components have been shown to have a promoting or inhibiting effect; they can raise or lower the incidence of a cancer that has already been induced by exposure to an initiator.

Dietary Guidelines

Despite the uncertainties about the role of diet in cancer, many scientists believe that sufficient evidence exists to recommend preliminary dietary guidelines for reducing the risk of cancer. After a two-year study of diet and cancer, a committee of the National Research Council (National Academy of Sciences) proposed such guidelines in its 1982 report *Diet, Nutrition, and Cancer.* In early 1984, the American Cancer Society began a campaign to urge the public to follow this diet.

The NRC committee recommended that the population reduce its consumption of both saturated and unsaturated fat from the present level of approximately 40 percent to 30 percent of total calories; eat fruits, vegetables, and high-fiber grains regularly; reduce consumption of cured, pickled, or smoked foods, which have been linked to cancer of the stomach and esophagus; and drink alcohol only in moderation.

These guidelines are, by necessity, preliminary. Given the current gaps in our understanding, there is no precise formula for preventing diet-related cancers. The situation is reminiscent of the uncertainty surrounding the role of smoking and cancer 20 years ago. If the population had been persuaded to stop smoking when the association with lung cancer was first reported, approximately 30 percent of today's cancer deaths could have been prevented. Many scientists, including the NRC committee, now believe that it may eventually be possible to define a diet that will significantly reduce the incidence of cancer in the United States. The next and by no means trivial step will be to persuade people to adopt that diet.

6

Dietary Carcinogens and Anticarcinogens

As epidemiological studies revealed numerous links between diet and cancer, efforts were increased to determine whether chemical mutagens or carcinogens occur naturally in foods. Epidemiological studies have focused on foods containing specific nutrients, such as protein, fats, and dietary fiber. Yet nutrients are only a small proportion of the chemicals that constitute various foods. Foods also contain many thousands of non-nutritive substances, as well as additives and natural and synthetic contaminants.

In recent history, food additives and contaminants such as chemicals used in food processing or residues of pesticides have engendered the greatest concern as possible health hazards. In the past two decades, many food additives have been tested for toxicity—although only a small number have so far been tested for carcinogenicity. Several laws and regulations are designed to minimize

---

This chapter is based on the presentation given by Bruce N. Ames, University of California-Berkeley, at the 1983 annual meeting of the Institute of Medicine.

human exposure to known or suspected toxins and carcinogens in food. The Delaney Clause of the Federal Food, Drug, and Cosmetic Act, for instance, prohibits the use of any food additive that has been shown to cause cancer in laboratory animals or human beings.

By contrast, the natural constituents of food have received much less attention. In the past 10 years or so, scientists have begun screening some of these substances, as well as some naturally occurring contaminants like mold toxins, to determine whether they, too, pose a cancer risk.

These biochemical assays have uncovered an extraordinary variety of naturally occurring mutagens and animal carcinogens in foods. In addition, some common cooking methods have been shown to generate mutagens. These studies reveal that mutagens and potential carcinogens are ubiquitous in the human diet—they can be found in celery, peanuts, hamburgers, and toast, for instance. Yet the magnitude of the risk they pose is not at all clear.

Part of the problem is the difficulty in testing. Because cancer is thought to arise from damage to DNA, substances that cause mutations are considered to be potential carcinogens. The first step, then, in testing a chemical is a mutagenicity assay. Numerous studies have shown that a chemical that causes mutations in any living cells, including bacteria, should be suspected as a human carcinogen and studied further. Lengthy and expensive tests in whole animals are necessary to prove that a substance is a carcinogen—even in that animal. Few mutagens in foods have undergone such tests.

Identifying a chemical as a mutagen or a carcinogen is only the start. Before its risks can be assessed, its potency must be determined—a difficult task when trying to extrapolate from laboratory animals to humans—as well as its prevalence in the diet and route of exposure.[1] Such work is just beginning on these natural mutagens and carcinogens. At this point, there is no evidence that any one of them is a major contributor to total cancer risk in the United States, yet a possible hazard cannot be ruled out.

---

[1] For a discussion of risk assessment, see *Risk Assessment in the Federal Government: Managing the Process*. Washington, D.C.: National Academy Press, 1983.

The picture is not as bleak as it may sound, however. A variety of natural foods have also been found to contain anticarcinogens—substances that inhibit carcinogenesis in laboratory experiments. The mechanisms by which they act are not known, nor is it clear if these chemicals have the same inhibitory effect in the living human body as they do in the laboratory. Nonetheless, the laboratory findings are intriguing in light of several epidemiological studies suggesting that certain foods protect against cancer.

In numerous laboratories around the world, efforts are under way to identify carcinogens and anticarcinogens in the human diet and to elucidate their mode of action. There is little conclusive evidence about how either might act to promote or inhibit carcinogenesis. One provocative—if quite speculative—hypothesis is that some optimum balance of carcinogens and anticarcinogens in the diet might act to keep cancer at bay, and thus by increasing consumption of anticarcinogens, it may be possible to prevent certain cancers.

Naturally Occurring Carcinogens

It is well known that certain molds produce highly mutagenic or carcinogenic toxins. The aflatoxins and sterigmatocystin, for instance, are among the most potent carcinogens known. Aflatoxin-producing molds are ubiquitous, but the toxin is especially prevalent in tropical climates, where conditions favor the molds' invasion of stored foods. In the United States, aflatoxins can enter the diet through crops that are invaded by these molds before harvest—usually peanuts, corn, and cottonseed, and less frequently, tree nuts such as almonds, walnuts, pecans, and pistachios. Other mutagens and carcinogens can be present in mold-contaminated corn, grains, peanut butter, bread, cheese, fruit, and apple juice.

Nitrate and nitrite are widely dispersed in the human diet. Nitrate is present in numerous vegetables, including lettuce, beets, celery, spinach, radishes, and rhubarb, in varying concentrations depending on the species, culture conditions, time of harvest, and other factors. In the body, nitrate can be converted to nitrite, which in turn can react with amines to form nitrosamines and other *N*-

nitroso compounds, which are potent carcinogens. Nitrite is also ingested directly, predominantly in cured meats. Tobacco also contains nitrosamines—the average smoker receives 10 to 100 times more nitrosamines from cigarettes than from dietary sources.

Nature's Pesticides

Plants synthesize a variety of toxic chemicals, which are used to ward off bacteria, fungi, insects, and other predators. For the past 100 years, organic chemists have been isolating and characterizing these plant chemicals: tens of thousands are already known, and others are still being discovered. Bruce Ames, the University of California biochemist who developed the widely used Ames mutagenicity assay, estimates that in general these natural pesticides constitute 2 to 10 percent of a plant's weight.

Despite the prevalence of these natural plant chemicals in the human diet, little is known of their toxicology. Only in the past few years have they been tested for mutagenicity or carcinogenicity. Many of them have been found to be mutagens, carcinogens, or teratogens—substances that cause birth defects.

According to Ames, these plant toxins can enter the diet in several ways, either by the direct ingestion of plants containing them, or indirectly, through the milk of animals that have eaten toxin-producing plants, for instance. The following examples, drawn from the work of Bruce Ames, illustrate the diverse sources of these naturally occurring mutagens and carcinogens.

Edible mushrooms contain a group of chemicals known as *hydrazines*, many of which are mutagenic and some of which are carcinogenic in laboratory animals. The most common commercial mushroom, *Agaricus bisporus*, contains several of these carcinogenic hydrazines or their breakdown products. The widely eaten false morel (*Gyromitra esculenta*) contains 11 hydrazines, 3 of which are known animal carcinogens. One of these is especially potent, inducing lung tumors in mice at a very low dose.[2]

---

[2] For more details on extrapolating doses from rodents to human beings, see *Identifying and Estimating the Genetic Impact of Chemical Mutagens*. Washington, D.C.: National Academy Press, 1983.

Pyrrolizidine alkaloids are present in thousands of plants, generally in nonedible species. In some plants, they are present in trace amounts; in others they constitute up to 5 percent of the plant's dry weight. Many of these pyrrolizidine alkaloids are extremely potent carcinogens, causing lung and other tumors in laboratory animals. Plants containing pyrrolizidine alkaloids sometimes contaminate forage crops and food grains, resulting in acute or chronic poisoning in livestock. They can also enter the human diet directly through the ingestion of herbal teas, comfrey leaves, and occasionally, honey.

Black pepper and oil of sassafras, used in sarsaparilla root beer and in other foods as a flavoring agent, contain *safrole*, an allylic benzene derivative and known animal carcinogen. Black pepper also contains a closely related chemical, *piperine*, in large amounts—nearly 10 percent of dry weight. There is limited evidence that extracts of black pepper cause tumors in mice. Tarragon and anise contain another carcinogen, *estragole*, which is also an allylic benzene derivative.

Celery, parsnips, parsley, and other members of the Umbelliferae family commonly contain *furocoumarins,* such as *psoralen derivatives,* which are potent carcinogens. One hundred grams of celery, for instance, typically contains 100 micrograms of psoralen derivatives. Moreover, the level can increase 100-fold if the celery is stressed or diseased. Celery pickers often develop skin rashes from handling diseased celery.

Because these plant chemicals are carcinogenic in laboratory animals, they represent a potential human cancer risk. The magnitude of that risk, however, has yet to be assessed. Numerous other plant toxins cause mutations in bacterial cells, which raises suspicions that they may be carcinogens as well.

Some of the most widespread of the known naturally occurring mutagens are *flavonoids*, which are contained in the edible portions of many plants. In the United States, the average daily intake of flavonoids is estimated at 1 gram. Roughly 25 percent of this intake comes from tea, coffee, cocoa, fruit jams, red wine, beer, and vinegar. One of the flavonoids, *quercetin,* is particularly prevalent in the human diet. Some data suggest that it is a carcinogen, others do not.

Glycoalkaloids, the chemicals that potatoes produce to ward off predators, are quite toxic. Indeed, two of these, *solanine* and *chaconine*, can be lethal to human beings at high concentrations. Different varieties contain varying concentrations of the toxic glycoalkaloids; one variety bred to withstand insects had to be withdrawn from use because of its toxicity. As is the case with the psoralen derivatives in celery, the concentration of glycoalkaloids can increase when the potato is diseased, bruised, or exposed to light. Some evidence suggests that solanine and chaconine may be teratogens.

Mutagenic or carcinogenic plant toxins have also been identified in cocoa, tea, coffee, mustard, horseradish, rhubarb, fava beans, and other foods or flavorings.

In addition, some alcoholic beverages, including Scotch and North American whiskeys, have been shown to be mutagenic in laboratory tests, but investigators have not yet identified the responsible component or components. There is also some inconclusive epidemiological evidence linking alcohol and coffee with specific cancers: alcohol with cancer of the mouth, esophagus, pharynx, and larynx; coffee with cancer of the bladder, ovary, pancreas, and large bowel.

Browned and Burned Foods

Two decades ago, several investigators reported that beef grilled over a charcoal or gas fire contained a variety of mutagenic chemicals known as polynuclear aromatic hydrocarbons (PAHs). That was one of the first indications that methods of cooking can generate mutagens. In that case, the mutagenic PAHs were derived from the smoke created when fat dripped from the meat onto the hot coals. If the meat was grilled so that it was not exposed to the smoke, PAH contamination was eliminated or reduced. PAHs have since been detected in a variety of cooked or smoked foods, including coffee.

In the past few years, it has been learned that many burned or browned foods are rife with mutagens and potential carcinogens. Much of the research was performed in Japan by Takashi Sugimura of the National Cancer Center Research Institute, and others. Several years ago Sugimura tested the charred surface of the fish his wife was grilling on their hibachi and found it was highly mutagenic. He subsequently discovered that the mutagens are created by the heating of protein—and the process can also occur during the cooking of other protein-containing foods, such as dairy products. Other researchers have found that mutagens can be formed in meats that are cooked at a normal, not a high temperature. Sugimura has identified nearly a dozen mutagens that are produced by the heating of protein or amino acids. According to Ames, roughly 7 percent of these substances have been shown to be carcinogenic as well.

The browning of starchy foods also creates mutagens, apparently through the reaction of amino acids and sugars. In the past few years, reseachers have found that french fries, toast, caramelized sugar, the crust of French bread, and other browned foods all contain highly mutagenic—but as yet unidentified—chemicals.

Anticarcinogens

Epidemiological studies suggest that some foods, including cabbage and other cruciferous vegetables and some components of dietary fiber, protect against cancer. The particular constituents responsible for these protective effects are not known with certainty. In laboratory studies, certain substances have been found to inhibit the process of chemically induced carcinogenesis. Some of these anticarcinogens, as they are called, are described in the following paragraphs.

Several vitamins are known or suspected anticarcinogens. In epidemiological studies, food rich in vitamin A or its precursors, carotenoids, are associated with a reduced risk of cancer of the lung, bladder, and larynx. (Vitamin A is present in liver and carotenoids are present in green and yellow vegetables.) These studies provide only estimates of vitamin A intake, however, and it is not clear whether the protective effects are due to vitamin A, the carotenoids, or other substances. Conversely, laboratory experiments have revealed that vitamin A deficiency tends to increase susceptibility to chemically induced cancers.

Some epidemiological studies show that consumption of foods

containing vitamin C (ascorbic acid) is associated with a low risk of cancers of the stomach and esophagus, although it is not clear which constituent of the foods is responsible. In laboratory tests, ascorbic acid can inhibit the formation of carcinogenic *N*-nitroso compounds, which suggests one possible mechanism for the observed effect. There is much less evidence to suggest that vitamin C can affect the action of already-formed carcinogens.

Vitamin E (tocopherol) also inhibits the formation of *N*-nitroso compounds, and there is some evidence that it can inhibit chemically induced cancers in the laboratory. Epidemiological studies are rare, however, because vitamin E is so prevalent in common foods, such as vegetable oil, whole grain cereals, and eggs, and thus it is difficult to distinguish its effect from those of other compounds in the foods.

The mineral selenium, which is present in seafood, organ meats, and grains, as well as in drinking water, has been shown to protect against cancer in laboratory studies and to a limited extent in epidemiological studies. In animal experiments, it inhibits the chemical induction of skin, liver, colon, and mammary tumors. It also inhibits the induction of mammary tumors by viruses. It is not known if or how readily this protective effect can be achieved at normal dietary concentrations; most of these studies were conducted using selenium concentrations far in excess of the normal intake, often at levels bordering on toxic.

Oxidative Damage

The mechanisms by which dietary anticarcinogens might protect against cancer are not known. Ames speculates that many antimutagens and anticarcinogens may act by protecting against cell damage caused by mutagenic forms of oxygen, such as superoxide, hydrogen peroxide, and the hydroxyl radical. Ames believes that these forms of oxygen may be a major contributor to the destructive processes associated with aging and cancer. It is thought, for instance, that ionizing radiation acts to damage a cell by generating the hydroxyl radical. Specifically, Ames suspects that they both initiate and promote carcinogenesis.

These active forms of oxygen are created as the by-products of normal oxidative metabolism, as well as by other ways. Because of their reactivity, these forms of oxygen cause abundant damage within the cell. They damage DNA, cross link DNA to DNA, or DNA to protein, and generally disrupt cell organization. They can also trigger the destructive chain reaction of rancidity, known as lipid peroxidation, within the cell. This in turn leads to the generation of additional mutagens and carcinogens, many of which are oxidants. (Oxidants increase the oxygen content of a compound by removing electrons and thereby increasing the compound's valence, or ability to react with other compounds.)

The body has many defense mechanisms to protect against these mutagenic forms of oxygen. Several enzymes, for instance, protect cells from oxidative damage. In addition, several molecules consumed in foods are antioxidants, substances that prevent aberrant oxidation and the generation of rancidity mutagens. Many of the dietary substances identified as antimutagens or anticarcinogens, such as vitamin C, vitamin E, selenium, beta-carotene, glutathione, and uric acid, are in fact antioxidants.

If active oxygen forms do prove to be involved in carcinogenesis, as Ames suspects, then one approach to cancer prevention may be to adjust the dietary intake of antioxidants, he says. At present, the optimum level of dietary antioxidants is not known, and excessive consumption of several of them, including vitamin A and selenium, can be toxic.

Assessing the Risk

As shown by the examples in this chapter, naturally occurring mutagens and possible carcinogens are widely distributed in the human diet. However, with a few exceptions, such as the aflatoxins and *N*-nitroso compounds, the significance of these substances for human health is not known.

In Ames' view, this recent—and continuing—detection of natural carcinogens in the diet will eventually require a reappraisal of health hazards and sources of carcinogens. The presence of pesticide residues in foods has engendered considerable concern and is aggressively regulated; by contrast, little attention has been paid to the intake of nature's pesticides, the plant toxins, says Ames.

He suspects that they may turn out to pose a greater risk than synthetic pesticides.

Additional research, including epidemiological studies, and long-term cancer studies in laboratory animals, will be necessary to evaluate the magnitude of risk posed by dietary carcinogens and mutagens. Before society responds to these potential threats, other factors will also need to be evaluated, such as the trade-offs inherent in removing these substances from the diet. Cooking fish or meat, for instance, does create mutagens. Yet cooking also destroys parasites and pathogenic microorganisms. Similarly, some plants containing mutagenic flavonoids are highly nutritious.

There are other possible implications of the association between cancer and dietary constituents. For example, in an attempt to reduce dependence on synthetic pesticides, some breeders are developing plants that contain higher levels of the natural toxins that confer resistance to insects. It may be prudent to determine which pesticides—natural or synthetic—pose the greatest health hazard, Ames suggests.

Questions of relative risk aside, it is far easier to minimize the occurrence of intentional additives and industrial contaminants in foods than it is to control the natural risk factors in diet. Historically, food safety regulation has tended to focus on such "foreign" sources of risk. Yet if it is determined that natural substances in the diet—major nutrients and perhaps these naturally occurring carcinogens—are the greater danger, then consumers may have to assume a greater share of the responsibility for protecting themselves. To explore many of the questions raised in this and the preceding chapter, the National Cancer Institute has embarked on an ambitious research program. Only when it is known which substances in foods either promote or inhibit carcinogenesis will it be possible to devise prudent strategies for preventing diet-related cancer.

7

Diet and Cancer: New Policy Questions

Since the passage of the 1906 Food and Drug Act, the task of ensuring the safety of foods has fallen primarily to the Food and Drug Administration (FDA). During this century, regulatory policy has grown incrementally with the passage of statutory amendments addressing one potential risk or another, such as food additives or the residues of drugs used in food animals.

In the past 25 years, FDA has specifically sought to eliminate possible cancer-causing substances from foods. The focus has been on exogenous chemicals—food additives, coloring agents, industrial contaminants, natural contaminants, and the like. In many ways, says Richard Merrill, dean of the University of Virginia School of Law and former chief counsel for FDA, the agency's strategy has resembled a "search and destroy" mission, in which FDA has attempted to identify and when possible remove from

This chapter is based on the presentation given by Richard A. Merrill, University of Virginia School of Law, at the 1983 annual meeting of the Institute of Medicine.

the diet those few agents thought to pose a cancer or other health risk.

In regulating potential carcinogens, the agency has been toughest on intentional food additives—e.g., the 1958 Delaney Clause prohibits the use of any additive known to cause cancer in human beings or other animals. Working with the Environmental Protection Agency, FDA has also set permissible limits for some industrial contaminants, such as pesticide residues. (However, the mechanisms for detecting whether a hazardous substance has inadvertently entered the food supply are weak, says Merrill, who cites the recent ethylene dibromide [EDB] episode.) In addition, FDA has set permissible limits for naturally occurring contaminants known to be carcinogenic, such as aflatoxins and other mold toxins. Throughout this process, the natural constituents of foods have received comparatively less attention. This partially reflects a longstanding assumption that foods that are grown and harvested are generally safe as long as they are free of additives and contaminants. It also reflects the feasibility of regulation: It is far easier to monitor and control the level of intentional additives in foods than it is their natural constituents.

Everyday Risks

The accumulating evidence about the relation between diet and cancer described in the preceding two chapters challenges some of the assumptions that underlie existing regulatory policy for food safety. As outlined in Chapter 6, recent studies suggest that a typical, everyday diet may pose a greater cancer risk than do food additives and contaminants, at least at current levels. In the past 20 years, epidemiologists have found that the foods people eat strongly influence the probability of their developing certain types of cancer. As described in Chapter 6, the high rate of breast and colon cancer in the United States and other affluent nations has been linked to a high intake of fats and fatty meats. Furthermore, frequent consumption of grains, vegetables, and fruits is associated with a lower incidence of colon, esophageal, and stomach cancers. Some scientists now believe that dietary factors may be responsible for anywhere from 10 to 70 percent of all cancers in the United

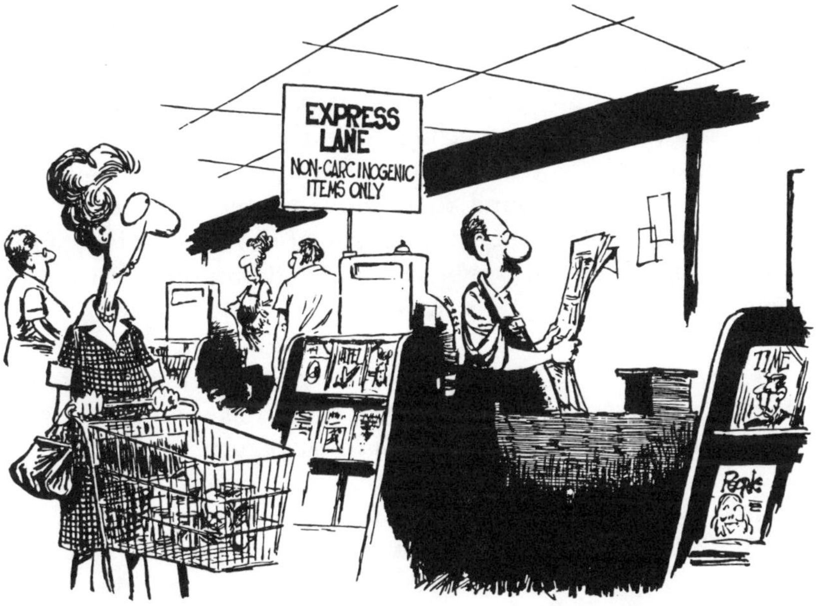

John Branch
(*San Antonio Express-News*)

States. By contrast, food additives are typically thought to cause at most 5 percent of all cancers, and environmental pollutants no more than 2 percent. These are preliminary estimates at best.

In addition, it has recently been found that natural mutagens and possible carcinogens are pervasive in a traditional diet. These substances have been detected in a variety of foods—including celery, potatoes, peanuts, coffee, cocoa, tea, and meats. Some of these foods—and vegetables in particular—also contain anticarcinogens, substances that seem to protect against cancer (see Chapter 6).

Self-Protection

Existing regulatory structures were not designed to address these new concerns, says Merrill, who thinks that as the scientific evidence strengthens, both Congress and FDA may need to rethink government strategy for preventing diet-related cancer. Diet now appears to be a far greater factor in cancer than was generally thought 80 years ago when the food safety law was written. Moreover, the problem is not specific, individual contaminants, as previously believed. Nor is it specific foods per se, as some of the dietary components found to promote cancer, such as fat, are essential nutrients. Rather, the probability of developing cancer seems to be influenced by the quantity and proportion of certain dietary components, and perhaps even by methods of cooking. In short, the problem is one of total dietary choice.

Indeed, two dietary cancer risks—too much fat and perhaps too little fiber—are associated with those choices over which the consumer has the readiest control. Yet past regulatory efforts have relied little on consumer self-protection; when additives and contaminants were considered the major hazards, the responsibility for prevention was thought to rest not with the consumer but with the government, which had the power to ban them.

This "pollution control" approach to prevention—the attempt to eliminate offending substances from the diet—may be outmoded, Merrill says. FDA will undoubtedly continue to regulate food additives and other exogenous chemicals in an effort to minimize exposure to carcinogenic substances. But given the plethora of natural mutagens and carcinogens, such regulations cannot ensure a risk-free diet.

For foods that cannot practically be eliminated from the diet, the government may be forced to rely on labels warning of potentially harmful constituents, as Congress has done for saccharin. Yet there are practical limitations to this approach. Fruits and vegetables are hard to label, for instance, and their characteristics vary both seasonally and regionally. Instead, FDA may be persuaded to resume regulating the composition of processed foods. In the 1940s and 1950s, FDA set standards for the content of cheeses, jams, mayonnaise, and numerous other foods. Such controls could be revived and modified to reflect new understanding of dietary risk factors, suggests Merrill. For example, FDA could set a limit on the amount of saturated fat allowed in processed foods.

However, this and other traditional approaches to control the characteristics of marketed foods may not be sufficient, according to Merrill. An additional and perhaps more effective strategy for preventing cancer may simply be to provide information that will help consumers make intelligent choices. And as the government's focus broadens from the control of the composition of foods to education, it may turn out that FDA is no longer the most appropriate agency for the task, Merrill concedes.

Several educational programs are already under way. Both the American Cancer Society and the federal government embarked on new efforts in 1984 to alert the public to the risks and benefits of certain dietary patterns. The federal cancer prevention effort, led by the Department of Health and Human Services, will focus on diet, smoking, and to a lesser extent, occupational safety. In the first year, nearly $700,000 will be spent on television commercials, pamphlets, and other materials. In addition, groups that have a commercial stake in what Americans eat will probably launch their own educational campaigns.

Personal Autonomy

Implementing such a policy will be a formidable task. Although it is relatively easy to eliminate contaminants in foods, it is much more difficult to influence dietary choice, Merrill suspects. The toughest obstacle will probably not be technical feasibility or cost, although a massive educational campaign could be quite expensive. Rather, it may be personal autonomy. People have an obstinate attachment to eating foods they enjoy, and they do not always welcome advice on how to change their diet. Moreover, even those individuals who choose to change their eating habits often have an extremely hard time doing so, as shown by the vast numbers of Americans who try perpetually, but unsuccessfully, to lose weight.

There are practical impediments to such a program as well. One is the complexity of the subject and the difficulty of translating the key information into accessible language. In addition, the potential for "information overload" is high, as FDA noted in 1979 when it was criticized for failing to require labeling of all foods containing possible carcinogens. Their response, published in the *Federal Register*, was blunt: "A requirement for warnings on all foods that may contain inherent carcinogenic ingredients or carcinogenic contaminants would apply to many, perhaps most of the foods in the supermarket. Such warnings would be so numerous they would only confuse the public. It would not promote informed consumer decision-making. It would not advance the public health."

The continuing scientific uncertainty also complicates the issue. While the weight of evidence implicating diet in cancer is strong, the associations between certain nutrients and cancer have not been proved definitively, nor have the biological mechanisms been worked out. Thus, consumers would be asked to alter their behavior on the basis of uncertain information. Moreover, because the data on diet and cancer are still open to different interpretations, the public may be bombarded with conflicting information as it was 20 years ago on the issue of smoking and cancer.

Determining the appropriate means of communication is another problem. Restaurant sales account for roughly 40 percent of all food consumed in the United States, yet FDA has no regulatory authority to require labeling or other information disclosures within restaurants. Similarly, large segments of the population, such as members of the military services or persons in various institutions, have limited choice about their diet.

Changing Habits

Perhaps the major impediment to an effective educational program is the paltry understanding of consumer behavior generally and dietary change specifically. Surprisingly little is known about the quantity and types of foods people eat, or the exact composition of those foods. Even less is known about why people select certain foods, or why they change their eating habits, as they often do spontaneously. At this stage, there are no proven methods for eliciting long-term dietary change.

This is not for lack of trying. Numerous studies have been conducted to assess the effects of nutrition information programs on dietary habits. The effect of saccharin warning labels on diet soft drink sales, for example, has recently been studied. Those investigators found that sales did drop at the height of publicity surrounding this suspected human carcinogen, but advertising also dropped at the same time. When advertising increased to its pre-publicity level in 1980, sales reached an all-time high.

Weight loss programs generally have a dismal rate of success. Very few people who participate in one of these programs are able to maintain their weight loss. There is some evidence, however, suggesting that a substantial number of people who fail repeatedly to reduce their weight can eventually succeed.

Perhaps most relevant to the diet and cancer issue is our experience with programs designed to prevent heart disease. In the recent Multiple Risk Factor Intervention Trial, a 7-year study conducted by the National Heart, Lung, and Blood Institute involving 13,000 men at high risk for heart attack, half of the group was given "special intervention" to help them reduce the factors that contribute to the risk of heart attack. Specifically, they were encouraged to stop smoking, reduce their blood pressure, and modify their diets to lower serum cholesterol. They did have reduced mortality from heart attacks during the study period. But the control group also modified these risk factors and had a lower mortality rate from heart disease, as did the entire U.S. population. It is difficult to evaluate how much of the change can be attributed to active intervention, how much to "spontaneous" change.

For over two decades, the American Heart Association has conducted an educational campaign to persuade the public to adopt a diet and lifestyle that would minimize the risk of heart disease. As the study described above and others suggest, many people in the United States have changed their diet and lifestyle in an effort to stay healthier. Moreover, mortality from heart disease has declined substantially in the past 15 years. It is not known, however, whether these lifestyle changes are responsible for the mortality decline, or in turn whether the lifestyle changes were the result of specific educational programs.

Although the underlying reasons for these changes in dietary habits are not known, they are encouraging. It may be that the public is responding to the growing scientific and medical consensus, communicated through many formal and informal channels, that diet is related to a wide spectrum of diseases, including cancer. Additional research may help in the design of more effective educational programs. Such programs will always be imperfect tools for preventing cancer, but as the accumulating evidence about diet and cancer makes clear, any effort toward prevention will have to emphasize consumer self-protection.

8

Cancer Medicine: Chemotherapy

If cancer is detected early enough, when the tumor is still regionally localized, the patient has a nearly 50 percent chance of being cured by surgery, radiation therapy, or a combination of the two. Unfortunately, of the approximately 785,000 patients who are expected to be diagnosed with serious cancers in 1984, only 30 percent will fall into that category. For the remainder, some 550,000 patients, by the time of diagnosis the cancer will have already spread, or metastasized, to distant parts of the body, or be circulating as malignant blood cells. New advances in cancer prevention and early detection may eventually improve those figures. Meanwhile, different therapeutic strategies are needed to treat those patients whose disease has spread by the time they are diagnosed.

Most of these patients will die within 5 years of their diagnosis. Once the cancer has metastasized, a surgical cure is impossible and

---

This chapter is based on the presentation given by Emil Frei III, Dana-Farber Cancer Institute, at the 1983 annual meeting of the Institute of Medicine.

radiation therapy is only rarely successful. Drugs may offer the best hope, for they can pervade the body and kill disseminated cancer cells when there are still too few to be detectable.

The difficulty, however, is that cancer drugs may produce adverse effects. Specifically, they are cytotoxic—they kill cells. The aim of chemotherapy—the use of drugs to combat disease—is to kill the cancer cells while doing minimal damage to the rest of the body. The strategy used for most cancer drugs is to target them to attack only cells that are rapidly dividing—the hallmark of a cancer cell. The antimitotic drugs, for instance, block one of the steps needed for cell division to occur. As most normal, mature cells divide slowly, if at all, they survive relatively unscathed. There are a few important exceptions, however. The cells in the bone marrow divide rapidly, as do those in the intestinal mucosa and the hair follicles. Hence, these tissues are also vulnerable to the effects of these powerful drugs. That explains the common side effects of chemotherapy—the temporary hair loss, nausea, and vomiting.

Since the first of these drugs was identified, clinical researchers have been attempting to strike a balance between their antitumor activity and their toxicity. In the past 30 years, they have made impressive advances in chemotherapy. Nearly 40 cancer drugs are now in use, all effective to some extent in treating cancer. In many cases, treatment has advanced from palliative measures that brought temporary remission from the disease to outright cures.

The National Cancer Institute recently estimated that some 46,000 of the 550,000 annual cancer victims whose tumors have spread elsewhere in the body can now be cured by a combination of chemotherapy and surgery and/or radiation therapy. The number may seem small, but only 30 years ago none of these patients would have had a chance of survival. For some types of cancer, the gains have been particularly dramatic. The survival rate for acute lymphocytic leukemia, a childhood cancer, has climbed from 4 to 60 percent since 1955, due largely to new chemotherapeutic regimens. For other cancers, however, few effective chemotherapeutic agents have been found. This is true for the most prevalent form of cancer, the carcinomas, or tumors that originate in the epithelial tissues. Surgery and radiation can provide effective treatment against a primary tumor, but when the cancer metastasizes, there is little hope of halting the progression of the disease. The search continues for new antitumor agents and new treatment strategies for these intractable cancers.

Trial and Error

The advances in chemotherapy have not come easily. The effort began in 1955, when Congress authorized the National Cancer Institute to start a Cancer Drug Development Program. From 1955 to 1975, some 40,000 drugs were selected annually for screening, largely on an empirical basis. Chemists looked everywhere—at synthetic compounds, fermentation products, and plant and animal products—to find those few compounds that might be able to destroy tumor cells. By the late 1950s, this process had turned up several promising compounds. Then the testing began. In a major clinical research effort, funded and integrated by the National Cancer Chemotherapy Program, numerous investigators began trying to determine if and how these agents could be used to slow the progression of the disease or arrest it.

In the early years, biochemists provided clinical investigators with agents that in the lab were capable of killing cancer cells. Yet it was at the bedside, in the clinical application, that the chemotherapy had to be proved. Largely through trial and error, the clinical investigators learned which drugs to give in combination and at what dose—an enormously complex question.

Soon after they began, the clinical researchers learned that cancer cells are notoriously recalcitrant. Indeed, the history of chemotherapy research is replete with disappointments and false starts. Some compounds worked well against animal tumors yet proved ineffective in treating human cancers. In other cases, agents that were particularly effective in shrinking tumors had to be abandoned because of their extreme toxicity. Later, when the clinicians thought they had developed a successful regimen and had induced a complete remission, the cancer would unexpectedly recur.

As clinical researchers developed successful strategies, they began to gain insights into the mechanisms through which these drugs acted. That knowledge in turn provided new hypotheses for the basic and clinical researchers seeking yet more effective agents and regimens. Gradually, as the understanding of pharmacology, toxicology, immunology, and cytokinetics increased, the empiricism of the early years of chemotherapy research gave way to a more rational approach. And all the while, the survival rate for some cancers continued to climb.

Childhood Leukemia

Much of the early work in chemotherapy was on a childhood cancer, acute lymphocytic leukemia, as well as on some of the other leukemias and lymphomas, which are malignancies of the organs that produce the blood, such as bone marrow and lymph nodes. In the mid-1950s, clinical researchers had three compounds that they thought might be effective in treating these cancers—prednisone, methotrexate, and 6-mercaptopurine. In terms of deciding how to use them, however, the investigators were starting from scratch.

They knew, for instance, that these three agents induced remissions in a minority of the patients who received them. Yet they did not know what the remissions meant in the context of overall treatment strategy—that is, whether remissions increased long-term survival. They soon found that those patients who achieved complete remission did have a substantial improvement in survival over those who did not. Hence, increasing the rate of complete remission became one of the major goals of chemotherapy.

To do so, the investigators began trying various chemotherapeutic agents in different combinations. The trickiest part was to determine the optimum dose. Generally, the higher the dose of a chemotherapeutic agent, the greater the response it elicits. Yet many of these drugs have their own dose-limiting toxicity—the dose at which they become too toxic to use. Consequently, when some drugs such as methotrexate and 6-mercaptopurine were given in combination, the dose of each had to be reduced to minimize damage to the bone marrow. These reductions took their toll in effectiveness; often two drugs in combination yielded little increase in the remission rate over a single agent alone. Fortunately, investigators found other agents such as prednisone or vincristine, a product of the periwinkle plant, which do not damage the bone marrow, and developed combined doses that in some cases were synergistic, that is, they produced a greater-than-additive increase in the remission rate. Combination chemotherapy was established.

By the early 1960s, researchers had designed a combination chemotherapy regimen to treat patients with acute lymphocytic leukemia that seemed certain to turn around their prognosis. While receiving this therapy, the children showed no signs of the disease; even examinations of the bone marrow failed to turn up any tumor cells. Hopes were high.

Unexpected Relapse

Yet before long, all of the patients suffered a relapse. Moreover, they often relapsed while they were receiving chemotherapy. "That was our first insight into the refractoriness of the cancer cell, which we now know to be specific tumor cell resistance," says Emil Frei of the Harvard Medical School and director and physician-in-chief of the affiliated Dana-Farber Cancer Institute. He and the other clinical researchers realized that they would have to continue chemotherapy during remission, a procedure known as maintenance, using still other agents to combat drug resistance. In addition, by adjusting the dose schedule—specifically by giving drugs intermittently rather than continuously—they were further able to reduce drug resistance and prolong remission. By 1965, the standard combination chemotherapy schedule for acute lymphocytic leukemia entailed one drug daily and another weekly.

As the investigators fine-tuned their procedures, an increasing number—90 percent—of the patients entered and remained in remission. Unfortunately, these patients began to show an increasing incidence of another cancer, meningeal leukemia. Sixty to 70 percent of them developed this disease, in which sheets of leukemia cells cover the meninges, the membranes that cover the brain and spinal cord. (The leukemic cells cause an increase in intercranial pressure, with associated symptoms such as headache, nausea, and vomiting.) The patients with meningeal leukemia then suffered a complete relapse of the systemic cancer.

Several investigators have determined how this second cancer arose. It seems that the meninges were already involved at the time the acute leukemia was diagnosed. However, the drugs used to combat the systemic cancer were largely unable to reach the central nervous system because they were blocked by what is known as the blood-brain barrier. Hence, despite a complete remission in the rest of the body, the leukemia cells in the spinal fluid or brain were able to proliferate and progress to a full-blown cancer. The problem was further compounded, it seems, because a minute amount of these drugs was able to cross the blood-brain barrier and pass into the central nervous system. Present in such a small amount, these drugs gave rise to a resistant cancer cell, which was then fed back into the systemic circuit, producing the total relapse.

In response to this new threat, the investigators began a treatment known as central nervous system (CNS) prophylaxis, which consisted of the injection of chemotherapeutic drugs directly into the spinal fluid, followed by brain irradiation. First they used conventional chemotherapy to induce complete remission of the systemic leukemia, then applied CNS prophylaxis. As a result, the incidence of meningeal leukemia dropped from 60 or 70 percent to 10 percent.

By 1965, the therapeutic approach was in place: combination therapy to induce complete remission, followed by maintenance chemotherapy and central nervous system prophylaxis. The survival rate for acute lymphocytic leukemia climbed dramatically. In 1955, these children had no chance of survival, and the median life expectancy at time of diagnosis was one or two months. By 1965, half of them would be cured of the disease.

The strategies learned in the work on acute lymphocytic leukemia have since been applied to patients with other cancers, such as advanced Hodgkin's disease and other types of lymphomas, again with remarkable success. In the last 10 to 15 years, the development and use of new cancer drugs has brought a cure rate of 70 to 80 percent for disseminated testicular cancer. Ten years ago, only 10 to 20 percent of these patients survived.

The Toughest Cancers

Unfortunately, the chemotherapeutic regimens that have increased the life expectancy for people with leukemias and lymphomas so dramatically have been less effective against the common epithelial tumors—the carcinomas of the head and neck, breast, lung, bowel—as well as melanoma, the deadly form of skin cancer. Investigators do not know exactly why these regimens are less effective against epithelial tumors. Some suspect that the different characteristics of the two types of cancer cells may be responsible. Those in the blood and lymph systems divide rapidly and are thus accessible targets for antimitotic cancer drugs. The epithelial tumors, however, are slower growing, which may enable them to survive these drugs.

Beginning in the 1970s, a group of clinical researchers worked toward a new strategy for these carcinomas, starting with breast cancer. For women whose tumor is limited to the breast, the cure rate from surgery or radiation therapy is near 80 percent. If the cancer has spread to the lymph nodes, the prognosis is quite different. In most cases, surgery and radiation therapy can control the primary tumor in the breast, but about 70 percent of the patients relapse within one to three years because micrometastases, microscopic pieces of tumor, have been carried by the bloodstream to distant parts of the body.

Chemotherapy is only marginally effective against a major, primary tumor. Research in the 1960s revealed, however, that the same drugs that are ineffective against a major tumor can be remarkably effective, even curative, against the cancer in its microscopic form. At first, chemotherapy had been used only after a relapse, essentially as a last resort. In the late 1960s, several investigators reasoned that chemotherapy might be effective if it were used immediately following radiation therapy or surgery to kill any disseminated cancer cells before they massed into a tumor. This approach is called adjuvant chemotherapy, and has been tested in clinical trials on women with advanced cancer who are at high risk of having a disseminated disease. According to Emil Frei, the results are encouraging, revealing a substantial improvement in short-term survival. Nonetheless, they are still tentative. In breast cancer, unlike most other cancers, the danger of relapse continues past five years. Several more years of observation will be necessary to determine the effectiveness of adjuvant chemotherapy in treating breast cancer.

Head and Neck Cancer

In the past five years, Emil Frei and his colleagues at Harvard have been trying to adapt the strategy of adjuvant chemotherapy to treat head and neck carcinoma. This is a particularly virulent cancer, afflicting some 37,000 people a year in the United States. By way of comparison, acute lymphocytic leukemia strikes 5,200 people a year. In nearly 60 percent of head and neck patients, the disease has progressed to the inoperable, and thus incurable, stage by the time of diagnosis, according to Frei.

The time-honored approach to these patients has been palliative treatment—usually radiation but sometimes surgery—which can provide a temporary remission. Borrowing a strategy used successfully in the 1950s to treat Wilms' tumor and some other childhood tumors, Frei and his colleagues decided to try chemotherapy as the initial treatment. Their hope was to reduce the primary tumor to an operable size or a size more amenable to radiation treatment. They call this neo-adjuvant chemotherapy, as opposed to adjuvant chemotherapy, which is used after radiation treatment or surgery.

In their first study, approximately half of the patients responded well to chemotherapy, enabling the use of surgery or radiation therapy to control the disease. Frei and his colleagues have since been trying to increase the response rate to this neo-adjuvant chemotherapy. They have tried various chemotherapeutic regimens, using different drugs in different doses given at different times. They have finally worked out a strategy, Frei says, that elicits an 80 percent response rate: in 80 percent of the patients, the treatment shrinks the tumor to less than half of its original size. Moreover, in 30 percent of the patients, there is complete tumor regression. In the first study, there were no complete regressions.

Although these results are encouraging, especially in these cancers that are the most resistant to chemotherapy, Frei cautions that this is only the first step. It will take several years to determine whether this approach will actually increase the cure rate for head and neck carcinomas and perhaps for other types of epithelial tumors as well.

The Future

Empiricism played a major role in the early years of chemotherapy. It still contributes—the recent recognition of the antitumor activity of platinum, for instance, was largely serendipitous—but to a lesser extent. Research in the past 30 years has provided a strong body of knowledge from which to draw. In addition, chemotherapy is increasingly influenced by advances in cancer biology and medicinal pharmacology. The methods of selecting agents for evaluation have improved, and the search is not nearly as random as it once was. Now some 15,000 compounds are screened each year, as opposed to 40,000 a decade or more ago. And for those agents that warrant further study, new modeling systems allow better preclinical evaluation of their anticancer activity.

As the recent work on head and neck cancer has shown, progress in chemotherapy has and will undoubtedly continue to come from the more imaginative and effective use of established agents. Advances in molecular biology have enabled investigators to determine the precise mechanisms of action of some antitumor agents. This knowledge can then be used to design more effective regimens. It also promises to provide insight into the differences between normal and cancerous cells.

Nonetheless, drug resistance and toxicity continue to plague chemotherapy. Investigations on a molecular level are beginning to reveal the biological basis of drug resistance, and new strategies are under development to combat it. In addition, investigators are learning how to modulate the activity of cancer drugs with normal metabolites (substances produced by natural chemical changes in the body), a promising approach to increasing the effectiveness of a drug while reducing its toxicity. For some cancers, it is already possible to treat effectively with little or no toxicity. For example, prostate cancer and some cancers of the breast are influenced by the endocrine system, and there has been some success to date in treating them with nontoxic hormones and antihormones.

Biotechnology also promises to have a profound effect on the treatment of cancer. Cells produce a number of substances, generically known as biological response modifiers, to regulate their own growth and to defend themselves against disease. A number of these may also affect tumor growth. As most of these substances are proteins, they can be produced through recombinant DNA technology. Several are currently being studied. These include growth factors and antigrowth factors. Perhaps the best known of these substances is interferon, the glycoprotein that cells release when they are invaded by a virus. Interferon increases the cell's resistance; the hope is to harness it and use it to combat cancer instead of viruses. Similarly, immunologists are beginning to understand the molecular basis of the immune system. The relatively new area of immunotherapy seeks to manipulate the patient's immune system to increase its ability to fight cancer cells.

Hopes are also pinned on another offshoot of the new genetic technologies, monoclonal antibodies. These are antibodies of unparalleled specificity, developed and cloned through immunologic techniques. It may be possible to target them to destroy specific cancer cells or carry existing cytotoxic drugs to only one type of cancer cell, leaving all other cells unharmed.

On a more speculative level, the identification of oncogene products—the proteins thought to be responsible for cancerous growth—may open up new possibilities for chemotherapy, such as agents that can destroy or interrupt the action of these proteins.

Both conventional research and biotechnology promise more effective, less toxic agents to treat cancer. The medical armamentarium is clearly growing, giving hope that it may eventually be possible to reduce the large number of incurable cancers.

9

The Psychological and Social Effects of Cancer

With the founding of the National Cancer Institute in 1937, the country embarked on a major program of cancer research. Clinical researchers developed improved radiation therapies, surgical techniques, and new chemotherapeutic drugs capable of arresting and even eradicating the disease in some patients. In the past 20 years, the 5-year survival rate for all cancers combined has climbed steadily. On another front, basic researchers have begun to unravel the biological basis of cancer—the molecular changes within a cell that give rise to malignant growth. Their work promises still more effective therapies to treat and cure more types of cancer, as well as new approaches to prevention. Now, after two decades of encouraging advances in medical research, attention is turning to the psychological and social consequences of cancer—the toll the disease exacts from the patient, the family, and the medical staff.

This chapter is based on the presentation given by Jimmie C. Holland, Memorial Sloan-Kettering Cancer Center, at the 1983 annual meeting of the Institute of Medicine.

Throughout the 1960s, there was a growing realization among the medical community that cancer care, to be effective, must address the emotional impact of the disease as well as its physical effects. At that time, the clinicians' understanding of these problems was based largely on observation and experience, not research. Some of the first controlled studies were undertaken in the early 1970s. Since that time, the field known as psychosocial research has flourished, attracting an increasing number of researchers and embracing new concerns.

The obvious starting point, when research began in the early 1970s, was to find ways to relieve the emotional turmoil of the cancer patient—the anger, fear, and the often debilitating depression. Since this work began, counseling and other psychological services have become an integral part of cancer care. Yet that is just the first step, according to Jimmie C. Holland, chief of psychiatry at Memorial Sloan-Kettering Cancer Center. Despite the increase in supportive services, she says, many patients remain seriously troubled, and additional forms of medical intervention may be necessary.

Moreover, other problems only now are being identified. Investigators have begun to examine the effects of cancer on the patient's family and medical staff—the depression, the chronic stress, the increased alcohol consumption. In addition, it now seems that prolonged or suppressed grief may have serious biological as well as emotional consequences, leading to an increase in illness and death among those who have lost a loved one to cancer.[1] And finally, there are special issues confronting the cured cancer patient. As the survival rate has increased, it has become clear that patients' troubles do not disappear along with the physical symptoms. The disease and the treatment may leave emotional scars that hamper the individual's efforts to resume an active, normal life.

All of these problems may be amenable to intervention of some kind—to counseling, education, or medication. Psychosocial re-

---

[1] For more on the health effects of grief, see Committee on Health Consequences of the Stress of Bereavement, Institute of Medicine, *Bereavement: Reactions, Consequences, and Care*. Washington, D.C.: National Academy Press, 1984.

searchers are now trying to understand these and other problems confronting the cancer patient in order to develop therapeutic strategies for relieving the burden of this disease on patients and their families.

Crisis and Resiliency

Cancer remains a terrifying disease. Fear sets in at the time of diagnosis and often persists throughout the ensuing months or years. On learning they have cancer, or that the cancer has recurred, patients experience shock and denial. They typically become anxious, depressed, or both. They lose their appetite and have trouble sleeping and concentrating. This "acute stress reaction," as it is known, is a normal, expected response to a crisis. Its severity and duration are somewhat difficult to predict, varying from patient to patient and influenced by many factors, including age, the site and course of the disease, the required treatment, and the level of support from family and friends. The reaction is usually self-limiting, subsiding to a more manageable level within a week or two. For some patients, however, this does not happen; severe depression and anxiety continue.

Holland and a number of other clinical researchers from several institutions have collaborated to study this and other problems. Recently, these researchers, known as the Psychosocial Collaborative Oncology Group, set out to measure the prevalence of severe emotional distress among cancer patients. Their yardstick was whether the patients were sufficiently distressed to warrant diagnosis of a psychiatric disorder.

In a study of patients in three cancer centers—The Johns Hopkins University, the University of Rochester, and Memorial Sloan-Kettering—they found that 47 percent were severely enough distressed to have a recognizable psychiatric disorder. Most were psychologically stable individuals suffering from a combination of reactive depression and anxiety, a transient but severe response to crisis, Holland says. Thirteen percent of these distressed patients were diagnosed with a more severe, or major, depression. For the majority, these reactions were directly related to their illness; few had unrelated psychiatric disorders.

On the positive side, says Holland, slighty over half of the patients were coping well with their illness, reflecting the "remarkable courage and resiliency of emotionally healthy human beings facing a major crisis."

Therapeutic Nihilism

This and other studies suggest that for almost half of all cancer patients, some form of intervention to relieve their emotional distress may be indicated. Many of the patients respond well to counseling; for others, antidepressants or other psychotropic drugs may be necessary. Yet remarkably few patients in the past have been given antidepressants, according to Holland. In a study conducted seven years ago, the Psychosocial Collaborative Oncology Group found that only 1 percent of the drugs ordered for 800 cancer patients were antidepressants. This reflects, in part, what Holland calls "therapeutic nihilism" among the medical staff: "The general feeling has been, 'Well, if you have cancer, of course you are depressed, so why bother to treat it?' " In addition, she says, physicians tend to avoid prescribing other psychotropic drugs and pain killers for fear that they will be abused. Holland has found, however, that cancer patients are "highly responsible" in their use of drugs.

Another factor in the negligible use of antidepressants is that they have generally been considered ineffective in treating depression related to physical illness. Holland and her colleagues have evidence to the contrary. They have found that certain tricyclic antidepressants, such as nortriptyline or desipramine, are particularly effective in treating depressed, withdrawn patients. For patients who have a mixture of anxiety and depression, the researchers have had success with another group of tricyclics, amitriptylin and imipramine, as these drugs have sedative and analgesic effects. Given these encouraging results, Holland suggests that controlled clinical trials be conducted to determine the effectiveness of these and other drugs in treating emotional disturbances related to cancer.

Different forms of intervention may be appropriate for other psychological problems. In some patients, for instance, part of the severe physical reaction to chemotherapy may be emotionally mediated. Chemotherapeutic agents can have extremely unpleasant side effects, including fatigue, fever, chills, and nausea. In addition to these effects, nearly one-third of patients receiving chemotherapy develop anticipatory vomiting, a conditioned, Pavlovian response: Just thinking about chemotherapy, or smelling the alcohol as they enter the hospital, is enough to start these people vomiting. For some patients, the anticipatory reaction is so severe that chemotherapy has to be discontinued. Antinausea drugs and counseling help, although in a recent study, the best results were achieved from a behavior modification technique known as desensitization, in which a person is exposed in small, cumulative steps to the feared object. This, too, warrants clinical trials, says Holland.

Chronic Stress

When the acute stress accompanying diagnosis subsides, it is often replaced by lower-level, chronic stress that lasts throughout the course of treatment. Patients are slightly more depressed than normal, slightly more anxious. They are often prey to sudden swings of emotion, alternating between moments of hope and despair. The physical manifestations are insomnia, fatigue, and loss of appetite, although it is often difficult to determine if these are stress- or disease-related.

The family is also subject to chronic stress. They, too, feel anger, fear, grief, and sometimes guilt over the plight of a loved one. And as they are coping with the illness, they often confront added financial burdens or perhaps greater responsibilities, such as child care. Moreover, their hardships often go unrecognized, as most of the attention and sympathy is directed toward the sick member of the family.

For both patient and family, individual or group therapy can help. In many parts of the country, there are special cancer groups in which patients can discuss their problems and gain insight, advice, or just sympathy from others going through the same ordeal.

The Physician

Most of these studies have focused on the patient, and to some extent, the family. Recently, psychosocial researchers have begun to consider the physician and other medical staff as well. The few studies that have been conducted to date suggest that oncologists (the physicians who treat cancer patients) may also experience chronic stress, Holland says, probably more severely than physicians in other specialities. They may describe the problem as "burnout," but Holland suspects that it is a reflection of the special emotional burden of cancer care, not just the normal, and by no means insubstantial, stresses a physician encounters.

A diagnosis of cancer is devastating to the patient. It can also be distressing to the physician, who often must convey this news several times a day. During the course of treatment, the oncologist must often give additional bad news and observe the suffering of the patient and the family. There are problem patients who have unrealistic demands, there are the tragic childhood cancers, and above all, there is the constant stream of deaths. Inevitably, some patients come to mean more to the physician than others, and the impact of their death is greater still.

These stresses may surface several ways. Physicians may become overinvolved, working long hours past the point of peak ability. They may become tense, irritable, and overly critical of the work of others. Or they may become uninvolved, detached from work, patients, and family.

They may also turn to alcohol or drugs. According to Holland, easy access to prescription drugs is an occupational hazard for physicians. A recent study by Steven Schreiber and Brian Doyle found that alcoholism is a problem for 8 percent of physicians; drug abuse, for 2 to 3 percent. Other figures are more disturbing: some 100 physicians, the equivalent of one average medical school class, commit suicide each year. Indeed, suicide is the major cause of death among physicians. It is not clear whether these problems are more pronounced among cancer specialists than among physicians as a whole. If so, special education and intervention strategies might be useful.

Cancer Survivors

Twenty years ago, the survival rate for all cancers was 25 percent. This year, nearly half of the individuals who will be diagnosed as having cancer will be cured. "Cured" is a difficult concept in cancer care: some tumors can recur after long periods of remission. It is hard to say with accuracy when an individual has been cured. Nonetheless, for most types of cancer, 5-year survival represents a cure.

By this definition, there are now some 3 million Americans alive who have survived cancer, and there are a total of 5 million alive who have a history of cancer but who have not yet had five disease-free years. These numbers reflect one of the great successes of contemporary medicine—of diagnostic techniques, surgery, radiation therapy, and chemotherapy.

Nonetheless, these patients' troubles do not end when they leave the hospital or when they cross the 5-year line. They are confronted by many medical, psychological, and social problems during the transition back to an active, healthy life.

Psychosocial researchers are now beginning to study the special problems of the cancer survivor. One of the first priorities, according to Holland, is to determine the delayed and long-term effects of both the disease and the treatment. For instance, a small percentage of patients develop secondary malignancies, a distressing consequence of radiation and chemotherapy. Research is needed to determine the prevalence of these secondary malignancies, how they arise, and specifically, how they can be prevented.

Both radiation and chemotherapy are relatively new treatments. Although their long-term effects on the body are generally not known, it is clear that both may damage the reproductive cells, leading in some patients to infertility. This is of particular concern, as many of the successful cancer cures have been for childhood and adolescent cancers. As these patients enter their childbearing years, they want to know about possible reproductive damage or risk. Few data are available at this time, although several studies are under way.

Similarly, there is evidence of central nervous system damage following some cancer treatments. In an effort to prevent a relapse in the central nervous system, many acute lympocytic cancer patients have been given cranial radiation and chemotherapy (see Chapter 8). Julia Rowland and her colleagues in the Cancer and Leukemia Group B in Scarsdale, New York, have recently found that the average IQ of children who received this treatment was 10 points lower than in children who received other treatments, but not cranial irradiation. Of course, damage must be weighed against the benefits of this treatment. In response to such studies of long-term effects, treatment programs can be altered to reduce undesirable consequences. For instance, in most cases today, the radiation dose used in therapy has been reduced, except for children at extremely high risk of a relapse in the central nervous system.

Fear of Recurrence

Many psychological problems relate to the patients' uncertainty about their physical condition and about the future. One of the most prevalent problems among cancer survivors, for instance, is fear of recurrence. This fear is deeply rooted in reality; physicians can provide no guarantee that all the cancer cells have been eradicated. Consequently, cancer patients can never be sure when they have crossed the line from illness to health.

Although the possibility of recurrence is always present, in some patients fear becomes excessive and debilitating. Some individuals feel extremely vulnerable, as if a sword is hanging over them, ready to drop at any time. These excessive fears are known as the Damocles syndrome. Fear of recurrence can lead to a debilitating preoccupation with the disease. Every cough, every ache is thought to signal that the cancer has returned. Some former cancer patients repeatedly seek medical reassurance. Others go to the opposite extreme, avoiding physicians entirely and neglecting essential health monitoring and maintenance programs.

Perhaps the best way to combat this fear is for physicians to provide solid information about the patient's chances of recurrence or secondary malignancies, according to Fitzhugh Mullan, who is both a physician and a cancer survivor.[2] It would also help, he

---

[2] Fitzhugh Mullan has written a book about his experiences: *Vital Signs: A Young Doctor's Struggle with Cancer,* New York: Farrar, Straus, Giroux, 1982.

says, to warn recovering cancer patients that they will feel these fears and that they are an expected part of the process of emotional healing.

Living With Compromise

Cancer often leaves a physical mark. Some patients lose a limb, a breast, a colon. Other disabilities, such as weakened lung capacity or infertility, are less visible. Adjusting to this physical compromise can be difficult. According to Mullan, the problem can be particularly severe for younger patients who are attempting to return to active lives that challenge their strength, endurance, and sexuality.

Again, education and counseling can help. Indeed, as early as the 1940s, the American Cancer Society sponsored a program in which patients who had gone through particularly radical surgery, such as the removal of a colon or larynx, counseled those who had recently been diagnosed as having cancers of those organs. Since that time, such programs have expanded considerably. Some of the best known are Reach for Recovery and Lost Chord.

For some patients, there is also the possibility of physical rehabilitation, such as breast reconstruction. In a study conducted with her colleagues at Sloan-Kettering, Holland has found that breast reconstruction can significantly reduce the emotional distress resulting from mastectomy and may help to overcome the reluctance of some women to have this life-saving but emotionally distressing operation. They found that the women who opted for breast reconstruction were psychologically healthy and well adjusted and had reasonable expectations about the surgery, realizing that it will not produce a truly normal-looking breast. Early concerns were that women who sought reconstruction would unrealistically believe that the reconstruction would solve other life problems, as is sometimes the case with other forms of plastic surgery. After surgery, most of the women—85 percent—were happy with the reconstruction even when the results was considered by the surgeon to be less than desirable. Perhaps most important, they were more satisfied with their sexual lives, had higher self-esteem, and took more pleasure in their appearance following breast reconstruction.

The Transition to Health

For the cured cancer patient there are social issues as well. As people make the transition from sick to healthy status, they have to confront the perceptions and reactions of friends, family, employers, and others. Families typically respond by overprotection; friends may tend to see the patient as someone special, either a hero or a victim. This "Lazarus syndrome" hampers a former patient's efforts to take up where he or she left off.

Cancer survivors may also be shunned by those people who are afraid or uncomfortable to be with someone who is or has been seriously ill. This reaction also surfaces frequently as job or insurance discrimination, according to Holland. Some employers are reluctant to hire someone with a history of cancer—even after a childhood cure. Some insurance companies charge former cancer patients a higher premium or reduce their coverage. One unfortunate consequence of these two forms of discrimination is that the individual becomes reluctant to switch jobs, and personal and career growth may suffer.

Bereavement

Despite the remarkable progress in cancer care in the past few years, slightly more than half of all cancer patients succumb to the disease. They leave behind family members who appear to be more prone to both physical and psychological illnesses. Some preliminary studies on the effects of grief have shown that both alcohol and cigarette consumption is elevated in families who have just lost a member to cancer, as is the suicide rate. A recent study by Knud Helsing and Moyses Szklo of The Johns Hopkins University found that widowers between the ages of 55 and 74 showed increased mortality rates from a range of illnesses, especially during the first six months after their wife's death. This increase in mortality rate was not evident in women of the same age group who had lost their husbands, however. Whether the increase in male mortality is related to a breakdown in normal health practices or occurs by some as yet unknown cellular route is not clear. "Research in this basic and common emotion—grief—is remarkably absent," Holland says. Similarly, little is known about the health effects on the oncology staff who experience repeated losses. Nonetheless, Holland and others believe that sufficient evidence exists to extend the concept of cancer care to the family and staff, as well as to the patient.

10

Alternative Care for the Dying: American Hospices

In the early 1960s, Cicely Saunders spent long hours with a friend who was dying of cancer in a busy London hospital. They talked often about the type of place where he would rather be during the last weeks of his life. The hospital, geared to treat acute diseases of the body, seemed cold, impersonal, and poorly equipped to handle the more chronic problems confronting a terminal cancer patient. He and Saunders envisioned a different kind of place, a special center for treatment of dying patients that would tend to the emotional and spiritual needs of the patients as well as the physical; that would relieve their pain, assuage their fears, and help them come to terms with dying.

In his will, he left Saunders, who was then a medical social worker, £500 to start a home for the dying. She went on to get her medical degree, then worked for several years in an existing

---

This chapter is based on the presentation given by David S. Greer, Brown University School of Medicine, at the 1983 annual meeting of the Institute of Medicine.

center for the terminally ill, called a hospice after the church-sponsored institutions of the Middle Ages that provided for the dispossessed and disabled. Finally, in the late 1960s, with funding from the National Health Service, Saunders opened her own center in London, St. Christopher's Hospice, and set about changing the nature of medical care for the dying.

Relieving Fear and Pain

She calls her center a home, not a hospital, and has described it as "high people, low technology." To counter loneliness, several patients share a room, which is typically decorated with family mementos and personal belongings. The hospice is open all day to visitors, and family and friends are usually in abundance. The intravenous drips, diagnostic machines, and monitoring equipment typical of a hospital ward are missing.

Dying is confronted openly. The hospice does not try to postpone the inevitable by heroic, and often traumatic, life-saving measures such as surgery or chemotherapy. Patients can be transferred to a hospital for such treatment at any time, however. Instead, the hospice staff, which includes physicians, social workers, psychiatrists, and a large contingent of volunteers, provides emotional support and concentrates on minimizing pain as the disease takes it course.

Indeed, pain relief is the hallmark of Saunders' approach to care for the terminally ill. She objects to the practice of giving pain medication only as needed, the standard hospital procedure that arose from fear of fostering drug dependency. By contrast, Saunders' approach is to try to prevent the patient from experiencing pain. In some cases, that means providing regular doses of the Brompton cocktail, a mixture of heroin, cocaine, gin, sugar syrup, and chlorpromazine syrup. Despite the often high doses, patients remain alert, she reports, able to face their last days without fear or debilitating pain.

American Hospices

Saunders' ideas spread quickly through England and Europe. The hospice movement came to represent both a philosophy and a system of care for the terminally ill. It reached this country in 1974, with the founding of the first hospice in Connecticut. The movement struck a particularly responsive chord in the United States; many health professionals welcomed hospices as an alternative to what they saw as the impersonality and overemphasis on technology of the American terminal care system.

In the following 10 years, hundreds of hospices were started in the United States; now some 1,000 institutions offer hospice care. Perhaps even more significant as a measure of their acceptance in the American health care system is the legislation passed by Congress in 1982, as part of the Tax Equity and Fiscal Responsibility Act (TEFRA), that provides Medicare coverage for hospice services.

It is the hospice philosophy, more precisely, that has taken hold; the exact implementation varies from country to country, and sometimes from hospice to hospice. In the United States, hospices have a decidedly different orientation from their counterparts in Europe and Canada. In most U.S. hospices, the concept of a homelike environment has been expanded to an emphasis on treating the patient at home whenever possible. By contrast, English hospices are principally inpatient facilities.

Even within the United States, hospices vary one from another in many ways. Some are affiliated with hospitals, some with home health care agencies such as visiting nursing programs; some with churches. Some are small, community-based programs, treating only a handful of patients, others are associated with large agencies that may treat hundreds. Those affiliated with hospitals often have inpatient facilities within the hospital, although they are usually decorated with homelike furnishings and are run by a separate hospice staff. Some of the freestanding hospices, unaffiliated with hospitals, also have their own inpatient facilities. Most do not, and instead are designed exclusively to provide care in the home, although they can arrange to provide hospital care if needed. Similarly, most hospices, including those with inpatient facilities, provide home care for those who wish to spend some time at home, or die there.

Underlying these differences in shape and size, however, is a common approach to care for the dying. As in England, U.S. hospices are used almost exclusively by terminal cancer patients;

only about 10 percent of hospice patients are dying from other diseases. (One of the qualifications for Medicare reimbursement under the new law is a prognosis of less than six months to live.) Care is planned and provided by a medically supervised team that consists of several types of professionals and paraprofessionals, including nurses, social workers, and volunteers. In all hospices, the family or close friends also play a major role in patient care. The hospice staff teaches the family how to care for the patient at home, and both family and patient are educated on death and dying. Support services are available to the family as well as to the patient, and staff members are available after the patient dies to help the family with their grief.

The prevention and alleviation of pain is a major goal of American hospice care, as it is in Saunders' St. Christopher's Hospice. Heroin is not used, as it is not approved for medical use in the United States. Instead, other narcotics and analgesics are administered to combat the persistent pain that afflicts nearly 50 percent of all cancer patients as they near death.

Assessing Hospice Care

In the past decade, many claims have been made about hospice care. Hospices promise better relief of pain than can be achieved by conventional cancer treatment, more emotional comfort and relief for patients and their families, and, given the reliance on home care and the minimal use of medical intervention, lower costs.

Only recently, however, has there been any attempt to evaluate these claims scientifically; to determine whether hospices indeed offer superior care for terminally ill patients. As momentum gathered behind the hospice movement, Congress in 1979 mandated a major study of hospice care. The National Hospice Study, completed in 1984, was directed by David S. Greer, dean of medicine and professor of community health at Brown University, and his colleagues at Brown. It was supported by the federal Health Care Financing Administration, as well as by the Robert Wood Johnson Foundation and the John A. Hartford Foundation.

For one-and-a-half years, the investigators tracked some 2,000 patients and their families as they moved through hospices and conventional care facilities, and analyzed data on over 13,000 patients. Specifically, the investigators tried to assess how hospice care actually differs from conventional care, what effect it has on the patient and family's quality of life, and its costs relative to conventional care. The study also examined the possible effects of Medicare reimbursement on the structure, staffing, and cost of hospices.

Two Types of Hospices

Although American hospices assume many forms, the investigators found that there are essentially two types: those with inpatient beds and those without. In the study, those with beds were called hospital-based hospices, regardless of whether the inpatient facility was in a hospital or not. Those without beds were called home-care hospices. The researchers studied a total of 40 hospices, comparing one type to another, and both types to 14 facilities offering conventional cancer care.

Ninety-three percent of the patients in the hospices had been diagnosed as having terminal cancer, and most of them died while in the hospice program. Over half of the patients spent a month or less in the hospice program; about 20 percent spent less than one week. Eight percent, however, remained in the hospice for over six months, some for as long as two years.

The investigators found a number of differences in the pattern of care patients receive in the two types of hospices. The most obvious difference was the site of care. As might be expected, patients in home-care hospices spent most of their time within their own homes. On average, home-care hospice patients spent only 5.2 days in an inpatient setting, usually in an acute care hospital. By contrast, hospital-based hospice patients averaged 18.2 days in an inpatient facility. Examined in another way, over 99 percent of the home-care hospice patients spent some of their time in the home, while that was true of only 67 percent of the hospital-based hospice patients; that is, one-third of all hospital-based hospice patients spent all their time in an inpatient setting. This trend was also reflected in the site of death. Sixty-two percent of those patients in home-care hospices died in their homes. By contrast, slightly more than 20 percent of the patients in hospital-based hospices died at home. These patterns have obvious cost implications, which will be discussed below.

Greer and his colleagues also discerned certain differences among the patients who entered each type of program. Those entering hospital-based hospices tended to have weaker family ties—for instance, they were more likely to live alone—and thus might have fewer relatives or friends able to provide home care. In addition, they tended to be more functionally impaired at the time of admission than are those entering a home-care hospice program. Nonetheless, Greer says, these differences are not sufficient to explain the different pattern of care the patients receive in the two types of programs. He concludes that care is determined largely by the structure of the hospice. "When they have beds, they tend to fill them," he says.

Medical Intervention

Both home-care and hospital-based hospices espouse a philosophy of palliative care rather than curative treatment. The study revealed that, indeed, during the last two to five weeks of life, hospice patients were significantly less likely to receive any kind of intensive medical intervention—such as radiation, chemotherapy, or surgery—than were patients in conventional care facilities. Hospice patients were also less likely to receive blood tests, X rays, and other diagnostic tests, regardless of the type of hospice (see Figures 10-1 and 10-2).

The investigators also looked at other clinically relevant aspects of care, such as the use of radiation therapy to reduce bone pain, or blood transfusions and other intravenous therapy to treat weight loss or hemorrhage. Patients in both conventional care facilities and hospices were equally likely to receive this type of radiation therapy. There was a major difference in the use of intravenous treatment, however. At all times, patients were more likely to receive intravenous therapy in a conventional care setting than in a hospice. In addition, that difference became more pronounced as the patient neared death: in a conventional care setting the use

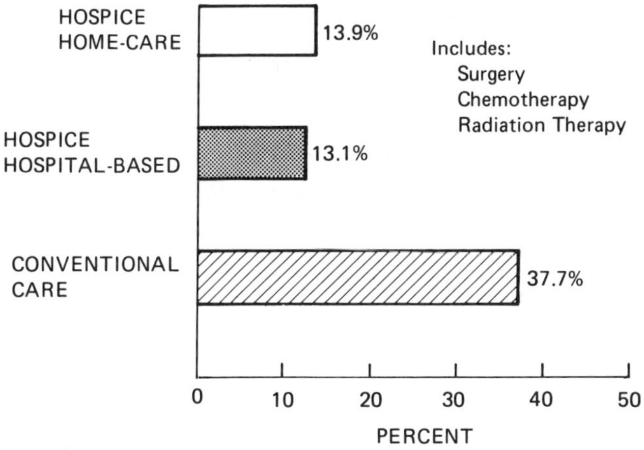

FIGURE 10–1 Patients receiving "intensive" interventions as last measure prior to death. (*Source:* National Hospice Study, Preliminary Final Report, 1983.)

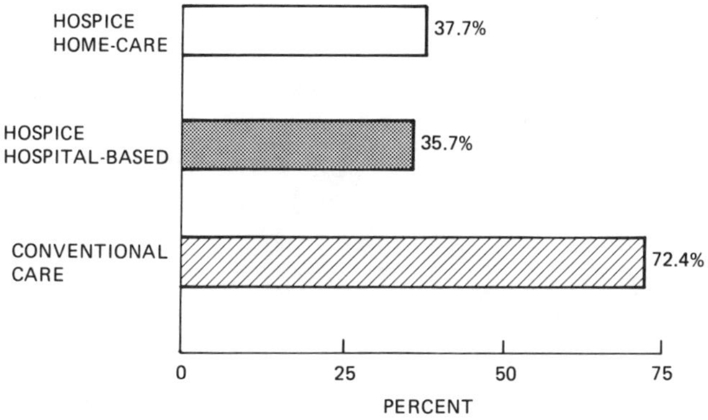

FIGURE 10–2 Patients receiving diagnostic blood tests, X rays, or scans as last measure prior to death. (*Source:* National Hospice Study, Preliminary Final Report, 1983.)

of intravenous therapy increased, while in the hospices it decreased.

By contrast, the percentage of patients receiving psychological and social services was greater in the hospices than it was in conventional care, reflecting the different allocation of resources in the hospice and the hospital. The same difference existed even prior to hospice admission, however, and may partially reflect the counseling that cancer patients received during the process of applying for hospice care.

Pain

About 30 percent of the patients in the study were free of pain during the last weeks of their lives. For the remainder, narcotics and analgesics were used in various combinations to provide relief. How well this drug therapy worked is difficult to assess. For many patients, the pain during the last few weeks was severe; many could not be interviewed during this time. Instead, the investigators relied on the judgment of the principal provider of care for each patient, for example, a family member. Their reports indicated that pain control may be better in the hospital-based hospices than it is in either the home-care hospices or in conventional settings (see Figure 10-3).

Given the hospice's objective of preventing pain, it was not surprising to find that pain control was better there than in a conventional hospital ward. A comparative analysis of the use of narcotics and analgesics confirmed that hospitals provided drugs largely on an as-needed basis when the patient is in pain, according to Greer. By contrast, a higher percentage of patients in the hospital-based hospice were on around-the-clock narcotics. What was unexpected was the apparent difference in the degree of pain control in the two types of hospices. According to Greer, a smaller amount of pain medication was used in the home. He suspects that families are reluctant to administer narcotics. As a result, home-care hospice patients received fewer and smaller doses of pain medication than did their counterparts in the hospital-based hospice.

Interestingly, the level of patient awareness was similar in the

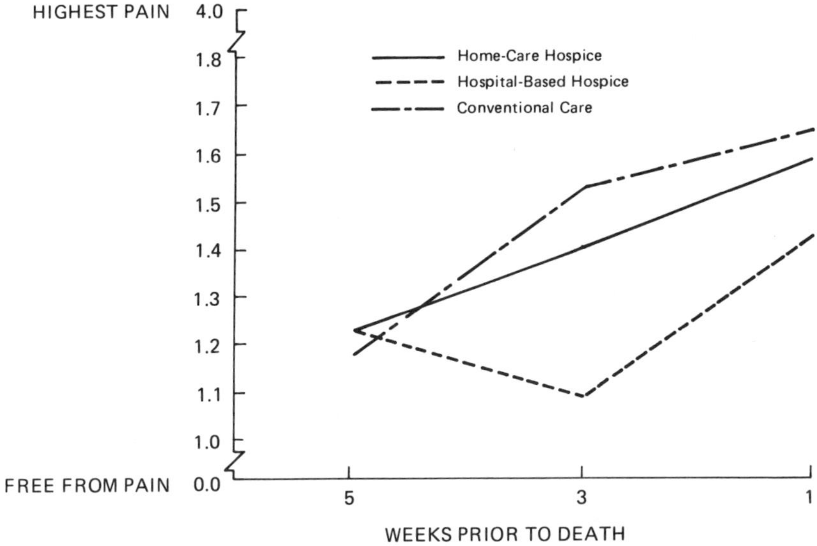

FIGURE 10–3 Mean score on pain index for "average" hospice patient as death approached. (*SOURCE:* National Hospice Study, Preliminary Final Report, 1983.)

hospices and the conventional facilities during the last five weeks of life (see Figure 10-4). In all three systems, awareness declined at roughly the same time, apparently regardless of the particular pain therapy received. This suggests that, contrary to many fears, pain medication can be used liberally without impairing functional abilities.

Quality of Life

Hospices strive to make the patient as content and satisfied as possible during the last weeks or months of life. To evaluate overall quality of life in the hospices and conventional care settings, the National Hospice Study investigators used several different indices that measured, among others, perceived health, outlook, family support, functional performance, loneliness, depression, emotional comfort, and patient awareness. Contrary to some of the anecdotal claims about hospices, they found that the quality of life

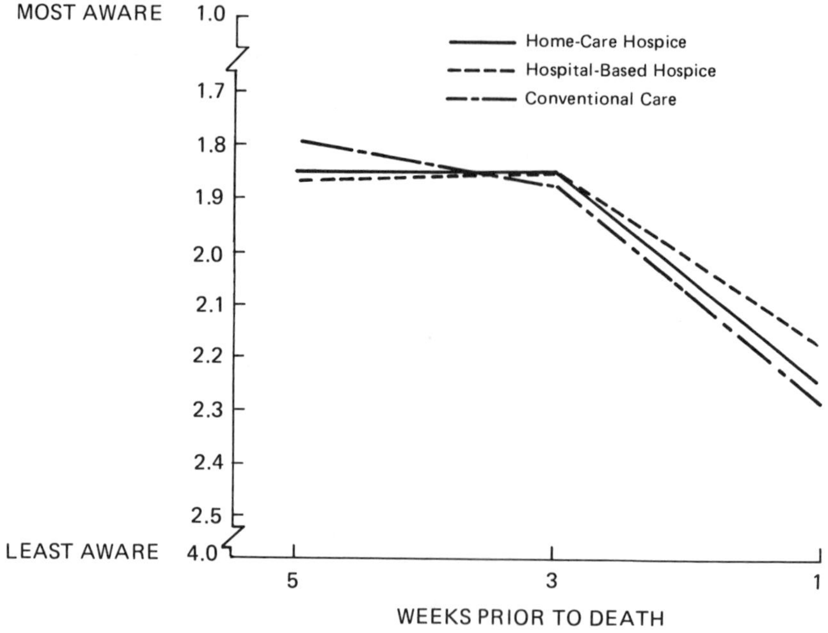

FIGURE 10–4 Mean score on awareness for "average" hospice patient as death approached. (*SOURCE:* National Hospice Study, Preliminary Final Report, 1983.)

was uniformly high, with no significant difference in quality of life across the three systems (see Figure 10-5).

They looked in particular at social involvement—contact with friends, family, and staff—because it is an important component of quality of life. Again, patients in all three systems reported a high level of social involvement. While patients in home-care hospices actually received more hours of instrumental care and visits, the reports of the primary care persons suggested that patients in the conventional setting had a slightly higher social quality of life than did hospice patients.

Similarly, although treatment varied significantly in the hospices and the conventional care facilities, all patients interviewed reported a high level of satisfaction with their care. Again, many could not be interviewed in the terminal period. The uniform satisfaction, regardless of which type of system the patient is enrolled in, may reflect preselection, Greer speculates: in other words, those patients who are inclined to want more intensive medical treatment probably stay in the conventional care system.

In addition, satisfaction with care was also high among the families of the patients, although it was significantly higher among the families of hospital-based hospice patients. The data indicate that home care is a significant emotional burden on the families. For the families of the patients in home-care hospices, the number of hours each member devoted to caring for the patient was staggering, Greer reports, and it appeared to take a toll on their well-being. There was a rise in illness among family members; in the first few months after the patient's death, the family made twice the average number of doctor visits. Nonetheless, despite the signs of strain, these families did not seem to regret their decision; they

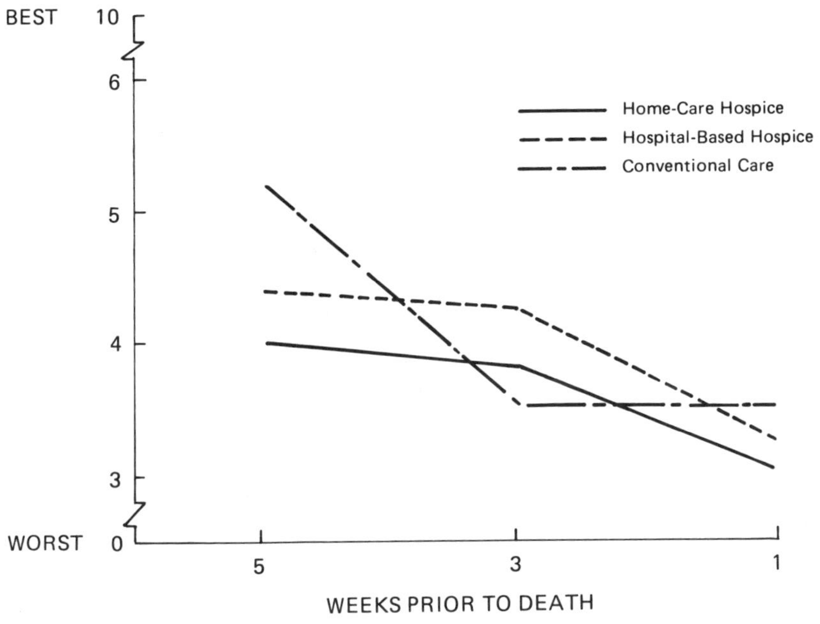

FIGURE 10–5 Mean score on quality of life index for "average" hospice patient as death approached. (*SOURCE:* National Hospice Study, Preliminary Final Report, 1983.)

derived great satisfaction from their ability to fulfill the wish of their loved one to die at home.

Costs

The recent TEFRA legislation allowing Medicare reimbursement of hospice care was predicated on the assumption that it is less costly than conventional care. The National Hospice Study investigators found that such comparisons are not a simple matter: patterns of utilization differ considerably between hospitals and hospices and between types of hospices.

For example, the average length of time spent in a home-care hospice setting was longer than the average stay in a hospital-based hospice. Further, when home-care hospice patients were hospitalized, the hospice had less control over the ancillary medical services. Consequently, the cost of inpatient care for home-care hospice patients was higher than it was for hospital-based hospice patients. For home-care hospices, the inpatient rates were $278 a day, for hospital-based hospices, $218 a day.

In total, however, because of their greater reliance on inpatient care, hospital-based hospices were more expensive than home-care hospices. The hospital-based hospice cost an average of $5,980 per patient; the home-care hospice, an average $4,758 (in 1982 dollars).

The major question, says Greer, is whether hospices offer a savings over conventional care. The study shows that hospices do provide significant savings, at least for typical stays of less than one month. For the last week of life, for instance, the cost of a home-care hospice was $910 lower, and a hospital-based hospice was $657 lower than conventional care. As the length of stay increased, home-care hospices continued to be less costly than conventional care, but hospital-based hospices became significantly more expensive than conventional care for stays above two months (see Figure 10-6). As mentioned earlier, the majority of patients spent fewer than two months in a hospice.[1]

---

[1] All dollar figures represent findings of the first year of the study and have been published in the *American Journal of Public Health*. However, the final figures vary from these no more than plus or minus five dollars.

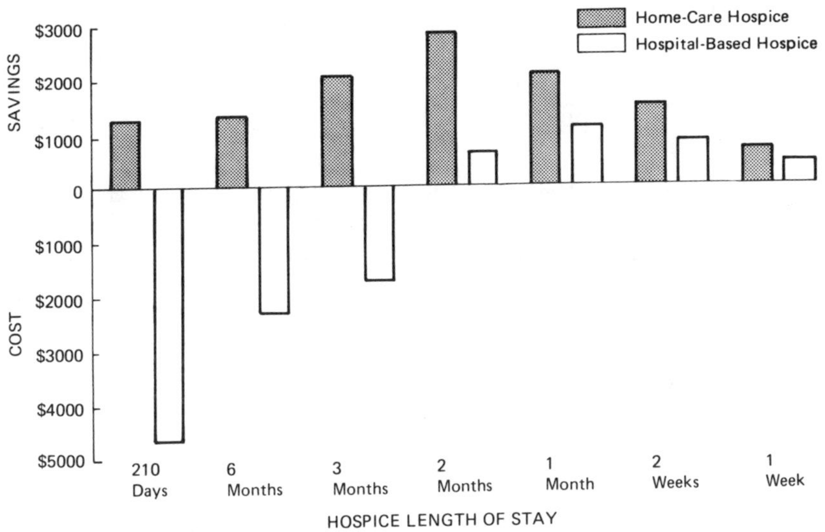

FIGURE 10–6 Cumulative Medicare savings/costs of hospice relative to comparable conventional care. (*SOURCE:* National Hospice Study, Preliminary Final Report, 1983.)

Something Intangible

Hospices do offer a different type of care for terminal patients. They are less likely to use intensive or heroic medical techniques, and are more likely to provide social services. There is some evidence that pain control is better in the hospital-based hospice than in conventional care setting, although such information is difficult to obtain from critically ill patients. However, despite claims of hospice advocates, neither type of hospice offers an advantage in terms of the patient's quality of life. It appears that the quality of life in a conventional care setting is not as bad as has often been portrayed, Greer says. Perhaps this reflects a recent and widespread shift towards a more humanitarian, less technologically intensive treatment of the terminally ill, he speculates.

For stays of one month or less, the hospice system can offer significant economic savings. Home-care hospices are less expensive than conventional care, even for longer stays. For that reason, the government might want to provide incentives to encourage the use of home-care hospices, Greer says.

He believes that both types of hospices are valuable alternatives to the conventional care system. Certain patients may be better suited to each type. For instance, patients with a high level of pain or weak family support may be better served in a hospital-based hospice.

Moreover, there may be other, less tangible benefits that were not revealed by the study, says Greer, who practiced community medicine 17 years before joining the university. During that time, he learned that many of the decisions made in medical care are based on "experience, impressions, and intuition," not hard data.

"Our study team spent many hours developing methods of measurement and inquiry designed to uncover all the salient elements of the hospice experience. Much of this agonizing was done in collaboration with hospice representatives. Yet as a man who has visited hospices across the length and breadth of the nations, I can say that there is something going on in them, something emotionally and spiritually inspiring and invigorating, that is not measurable using current techniques and that cannot even be described, except perhaps by the best of our poets."

Medicare reimbursement will make hospice care available to a wider number of people. Yet government participation, which means new federal regulations and restrictions, will also increase administrative costs and the complexity of management, perhaps driving out the volunteer-dominated community hospices. "Their loss would have a great impact on the hospice movement, both philosophically and programmatically," Greer says. Restrictions in Medicare reimbursement may prompt hospices to change their structure or policies, for instance, by increasing the numbers of short-stay patients.

In the face of increasing regulation, Greer says, the overriding challenge to the hospice system will be to maintain those elusive elements that make hospices unique.

Glossary

AMINO ACID Any of a group of organic acids that are the building blocks of proteins.

B-CELL Subgroup of cells produced in the lymph system, responsible for secreting circulating antibodies.

CARCINOGENESIS Multistep process of abnormal cell growth culminating in cancer.

CARCINOMA Malignant tumor derived from epithelial tissue (outermost covering or lining of all free surfaces of the body); may be composed of undifferentiated cells or may closely resemble normal tissue.

CAROTENOIDS Fat-soluble, yellow-to-orange/red pigments universally present in the photosynthetic tissues of algae, photosynthesizing bacteria, and eukaryotic—containing cells with a well-defined nucleus—plants; believed to be anticarcinogenic either in themselves or through their conversion product, vitamin A.

CELL LINE A mass of genetically identical cells grown from an originating cell in a culture medium under laboratory conditions.

CODON The basic unit of the genetic code. Each codon, a sequence of three nucleotide bases in a gene, is translated into one amino acid during protein biosynthesis.

CRUCIFEROUS VEGETABLES Members of the mustard family (Cruciferae), including broccoli, cabbage, cauliflower, brussels sprouts, kohlrabi, and turnips; in their raw form believed to protect against colorectal cancer.

GENOME An organism's entire complement of DNA, which determines its genetic makeup.

INITIATION The first step of carcinogenesis; takes place at the molecular level.

LEUKEMIA Any one of a complex of malignant diseases, chronic or acute, marked by an excess number of one of the types of white blood cells (leukocytes): lymphocytes, produced in the lymph nodes and spleen; granulocytes, produced in the bone marrow; or monocytes, produced in the connective tissue.

LYMPHOMA Malignant growth of lymphocytes. Abnormal cells may disseminate in the blood or remain localized in lymph nodes.

METASTASIS The spread of individual cancerous cells of a tumor from their primary site. Metastasized cells may remain disseminated (as in leukemia and some lymphomas) or colonize into new tumors.

MITOSIS The process by which the nucleus of a cell (in which the DNA has replicated itself) divides, such that two daughter cells are produced with the same number of chromosomes as the parent cells.

MONOCLONAL ANTIBODIES Highly specific and pure antibodies, obtained through the use of recombinant DNA technology, that attach to individual sites on the surface of a protein.

MUTAGEN A physical or chemical agent capable of inducing a mutation.

MUTATION In genetics and molecular biology: a sudden change, either in the base sequence of DNA or in the order, number, or placement of genes on or across chromosomes, that may result in a change in the structure or function of a protein.

NEUROBLASTOMA Malignant tumor characterized by immature, only slightly differentiated nerve cells of embyronic type.

NUCLEOTIDE Subunit of DNA or RNA consisting of a sugar molecule, a phosphate molecule, and one of four possible base molecules: adenine, thymine, guanine, or cytosine (in RNA another base, uracil, is found instead of thymine).

POINT MUTATION Change in a single nucleotide base, which can alter the message of a codon. This in turn can cause a change in the order of assembled amino acids, resulting in synthesis of an altered or completely different protein.

PROMOTER In carcinogenesis: a chemical that increases the carcinogenic activity of other agents that initiate carcinogenesis. In genetics: a region of DNA that is the initial binding site for the enzyme that will transcribe a gene into RNA.

PSYCHOTROPIC DRUG Any of a broad category of drugs, the primary action of which causes a marked and usually predictable change in mental state; includes tranquilizers, stimulants, antidepressants, barbiturates, and hallucinogens.

RECOMBINANT DNA TECHNOLOGY The methodology and techniques involved in forming hybrid molecules under laboratory conditions by splicing segments of DNA and rejoining them in a novel arrangement.

REPLICATION Refers to both self-synthesis of DNA and synthesis of RNA by DNA. In the latter case, single-stranded DNA serves as a template for RNA. DNA reproduces itself by separating into two strands, each of which then synthesizes a complement of itself.

RETROVIRUS Any of a class of viruses the genetic material of which is RNA instead of DNA. All viruses must use the genetic machinery of a host cell to reproduce themselves, but retroviruses undergo an extra step in which RNA is copied into DNA.

SARCOMA Malignant tumor, poorly differentiated, derived from connective tissue such as blood, bone, and cartilage.

TERATOGEN A physical or chemical agent that causes a birth defect.

TRANSCRIPTION The first step of protein biosynthesis, in which DNA directs the production of RNA.

TRANSLATION The second step of protein biosynthesis, in which RNA directs the assembling of amino acids to form the primary structures of proteins.

TRANSLOCATION Movement of a gene or genes from one chromosome to another (includes the exchange of genes between chromosomes).

TUMORIGENESIS The induction of a benign or malignant growth of abnormal cells.

Index

A

acute lymphocytic leukemia, 11, 82–86, 88, 98
adenine, 33
  see also TAT
adjuvant chemotherapy, *see under* chemotherapy
aflatoxins, 65, 71, 74
Africa, 40, 53, 54
Agaricus bisporus, 66
age, 4, 49, 55, 56, 58, 70
alcohol, 55, 61, 68, 92, 96
alleles, 45, 46
allylic benzenes, 67
almonds, 65
American Cancer Society, 60, 77, 99
American Heart Association, 79
Ames, Bruce, 63, 66, 69, 70, 71–72
Ames mutagenicity assay, 66
amines, 65
amino acids, 25, 33, 34–35, 69
  see also proteins; *and specific amino acids*
amitriptylin, 94
analgesics, 92, 95, 106
anger, 14, 94
aniline dye, 50
animal tumor cells, 18–19
anise, 67
antibodies and antibiotics, 12, 13, 40, 41, 42, 43, 46, 90
anticarcinogens, 10, 69–72, 75
antidepressants, 94
antigens, 12
antigrowth factors, 90
antihormones, 90
antimitotic cancer drugs, 82, 87
antinausea drugs, 95
antioxidants, 71
antitumor agents, 12, 82, 89
anxiety, 14, 93, 94, 95

appetite, loss of, 95
apple juice, 65
Armstrong, Bruce, 55–56
ascorbic acid, *see* vitamin C
Asia, 53, 54
Astrin, Susan M., 23

B

B-cells, 40, 41, 44, 46
bacteria, 66, 67
Barbacid, Mariano, 29, 30, 33–36
Battey, Jim, 44
beef, 54, 58, 68
beer, 67
beets, 65
bereavement, 100–101
beta-carotene, 71
beverages, 10
  see also specific beverages
Billeter, Martin, 20
biochemistry and biochemists, 6, 7, 24, 27, 32, 35, 36, 64, 83
biology and biologists, 1, 6–8, 17–18, 23, 39, 46, 89, 90, 91
  see also molecular biology and biologists
biotechnology, 90
birth defects, 66
Bishop, J. Michael, 19, 21
black pepper, 67
blacks, 2, 58
bladder cancer, 5, 23, 30, 31, 50, 51, 56, 68, 69
blood and bloodstream, 5, 6, 26, 84, 87, 108, 109
blood-brain barrier, 86
blood pressure, 79
Blym, 46
bone marrow, 5, 11, 82, 84, 85
bowel cancer, 12
brain, 85, 86
bran, 59
bread, 54, 55
breast cancer, 4, 5, 12, 17, 31, 52, 53–54, 55, 56, 57–58, 59, 70, 74, 87–88, 90, 99
breast reconstruction, 99
Broca, Pierre Paul, 17
broccoli, 59
Brompton cocktail; 104
Brugge, Joan B., 24
brussels sprouts, 59
Burkitt lymphoma, 32, 40–47

C

c-*myc* genes, 21, 23
c-*src* genes, 21
cabbage, 59
California, 58
calories and caloric intake, 59, 61
Canada, 53, 54, 56, 57, 58, 105
cancer
  adolescent, 97
  anxiety and, 14, 93, 94, 95
  bereavement and, 100–101
  biology of, 6–8
  bladder, 5, 24, 30, 31, 50, 51, 56, 68, 69
  bowel, 12
  breast, 4, 5, 12, 17, 31, 52, 53–54, 55, 56, 57–58, 59, 70, 74, 87–88, 90, 99
  central nervous system and, 97–98
  cervical, 12, 56
  chemicals and, 6, 8, 9, 10, 19, 21, 23, 30, 36, 50, 51, 59, 60, 63–72, 73, 76
  chemotherapy and, 6, 11–12, 14, 81–90, 91, 95, 97, 98
  childhood, 11, 82–86, 96, 97
  chromosomes and, 8, 18, 19, 39, 47
  cigarette smoking and, 9, 10, 36, 50–51, 52, 55, 61, 66, 77, 78
  colon, 4, 5, 31, 52, 53, 54, 56, 58–59, 70, 74, 99
  colorectal, 53–54, 55, 56, 57, 58–59

counseling and, 92, 99
cure rates for, 1, 5, 11, 12, 81, 82, 86, 87, 89, 92, 97
death rates for, 4, 5, 12
depression and, 14, 92, 93, 94, 95, 111
diet and, 6, 8–11, 49–61, 63–72, 73–80
drugs and, 6, 11–12, 13, 14, 15, 81–90, 91, 94, 96, 110
early detection of, 12–13
education and, 92, 99
emotional aspects of, 14, 91–101, 106, 111–114
environment and, 8, 9, 15, 36, 50, 74
epithelial, 12, 87
esophageal, 61, 68, 70, 74
ethnic origin and, 50
fats and, 9, 55–57, 59, 61, 63, 68, 74, 76
fear of, 14, 92, 93, 95, 98–99, 104
fibers and, 9, 58, 59, 61, 63, 69, 76
foods and, 9, 51–52, 68–69, 73–80
gastric, 56
gastrointestinal, 55
global patterns and, 50
hazards, 64
head and neck, 12, 88–89
heredity and, 9
hospices and, 14, 103–116
hospitals and, 1, 97
implications of, 14–15
intestinal, 56
kidney, 51, 56
large bowel, 68
laryngeal, 68, 69, 99
lifestyle and, 9, 50, 51
lip, 56
liver, 5, 70
lung, 4, 5, 9, 12, 31, 50, 51, 67, 69, 99
medical aspects of, 11–12, 13–14, 81–90, 92
migrants and, 50, 53–54
minerals and, 10, 70
mouth, 68
neck, *see* cancer, head and neck
nutrients and, 9, 10, 57, 59, 63, 78
nutrition and, 6, 55, 78, 79
oncogenes and, 6–8, 12, 15, 18–26, 29, 37, 39–47, 90
oral, 4
ovarian, 4, 56, 68
pancreatic, 4, 5, 51, 56, 68
patients, psychosocial effects of cancer on, 13–14, 91–101, 110, 111–114
patients, psychosocial effects of cancer on families of, 14, 91–101, 111–114
patients, psychosocial effects of cancer on medical staff of, 14, 91–101, 111–114
patients, psychosocial effects of cancer on physicians of, 96
pesticides and, 10, 63, 66, 68, 71, 74
prevention of, 1, 6, 10–11, 15, 27, 65, 71, 76
prostate, 4, 5
proteins and, 6–8, 12, 18, 63, 69, 90
psychosocial aspects of, 6, 13–14, 91–101
radiation and, 6, 7, 8, 13, 14, 15, 19, 21, 23, 30, 70, 81–82, 88, 91, 97, 98
rectal, 4, 5, 53, 56, 59
recurrence of, 13, 83, 98, 99
relapses in, 85–88
religious groups and, 55
remission of, 82, 84, 85, 86, 88
renal, 56
research laboratories and, 1
risk, 9, 10, 51, 52, 56, 60, 64, 67, 70, 71–72, 74–75, 76, 77
scrotal, 50
skin, 70
stomach, 4, 5, 61, 70, 74

stress and, 14, 92, 93, 95, 96
surgery and, 13, 15, 81–82, 87, 88, 97, 99
survivors and survival rates for, 1, 2, 3, 12–13, 84, 86, 87, 91, 97–98, 100
testicular, 56, 86
tobacco and, 4, 6, 9
transition to health and, 100
treatment of, 1, 6, 12–14, 27, 81–90, 97–98, 103–116
urinary, 4
uterine, 4, 5, 52, 56
viruses and, 7, 8, 9, 18–24, 29, 30, 31, 40, 46, 49, 50, 70, 90
vitamins and, 69–70
Cancer Drug Development Program, 83
caramelized sugar, 69
carbohydrates, 26
carcinogens and carcinogenesis, 4, 7, 8–10, 11–12, 20, 21, 26–27, 30, 31, 32, 36, 46–47, 59, 60, 63–64, 71–72, 74, 75, 78, 79, 82, 87, 88
see also mutagens and mutagenesis; tumors and tumorigenesis
carcinomas, *see* carcinogens and carcinogenesis; tumors and tumorigenesis
Caribbeans, 58
carotenoids, 69
Carroll, Kenneth, 56
case-control studies, 57–59
CAT scan, 13
Caucasians, *see* whites
cauliflower, 59
celery, 64, 65, 67, 68, 75
cell culture assay, 32
cells
abnormal, 5, 7, 6–8, 11–12, 20
animal, 6, 18, 21, 29, 30
cultures, 22, 26, 32, 44, 59
differentiation of, 5, 17, 22, 32, 60
division of, 17, 19, 45, 46, 82
growth of, 5–6, 12, 17, 19, 25, 30, 32, 45, 46, 90
human, 6, 8, 18, 29, 30, 31
leukemia, 11, 85–86
mammalian, 32
mutation of, 5, 19, 31, 64, 67
normal, 6–8, 11, 18, 19, 21, 22, 24, 25, 31, 32, 36, 43, 82, 89
oncogenes and, 6–8, 12, 15, 18–26, 29–37
proliferation of, 60
proteins and, 18, 19, 20, 24–26, 43, 44, 71
reproductive, 97
transformed, 6, 20, 22, 26, 30, 32–33, 46
cellulose, 58, 59
central nervous system, 86, 97–98
central nervous system (CNS) prophylaxis, 86
see also chemotherapy
cereals, 70
cervical cancer, 12, 56
chaconine, 68
charcoal, 68
cheeses, 65, 76
chemicals, 6, 7, 8, 9, 19, 21, 23, 30, 36, 49, 51, 59, 60, 63–72, 73, 76
see also chemotherapy
chemotherapy
adjuvant, 88
advances in, 11–12, 83
breast cancer and, 87–88
cancer and, 6, 11–12, 14, 81–90, 91, 97, 98
childhood leukemia and, 84–85
combination, 86
future of, 6, 89–90
head and neck cancer and, 88–89
immunotherapy and, 90
maintenance, 86
neo-adjuvant, 88
radiation therapy and, 14, 87, 88
reactions to, 95
relapses and, 85, 86

surgery and, 87, 88
trial and error in use of, 11, 83, 84
childhood leukemia, 11, 82–86
chills, 95
chlorpromazine syrup, 104
cholesterol, 57
see also fats
chromosomes, 8, 18, 19, 23, 39–47
see also genes
cigarette smoking, 9, 10, 36, 50–51, 52, 55, 61, 66, 77, 78, 79
clinical research, 13, 82, 83–84, 85–88, 91–101
cocaine, 104
cocoa, 67, 68, 75
Cochran, Brent, 45
codon, 33, 34
coffee, 55, 67, 68, 75
Coffin, John M., 20
Cole, Michael, 42
Collett, Marc S., 25
colon cancer, 4, 5, 31, 52, 53, 54, 56, 58, 59, 70, 74, 99
colorectal cancer, 53–54, 55, 56, 57, 58–59
coloring agents, 73
comfrey, 67
computerized axial tomograph, *see* CAT scan
Congress, U.S., *see* U.S. Congress
Connecticut, 105
consumer self-protection, 75–80
contaminants, 9, 10, 63, 64, 68, 72, 73, 74, 76, 77
Cooper, Geoffrey M., 30
corn, 8, 65
cottonseed, 65
Croce, Carlo, 42, 43
cruciferous vegetables, 59
cure rates, for cancer, 1, 5, 11, 12, 81, 82, 86, 87, 89, 92, 97
cytokinetics, 84
cytotoxins and cytotoxic drugs, 12, 82, 90

D

dairy products, 69
Dalla-Favera, Ricardo, 36, 42
Damocles syndrome, 98
death rates, for cancer, 4, 5, 12
Delaney Clause, of Food, Drug, and Cosmetic Act, 64, 74
Della Porta, Guiseppe, 36
deoxyribonucleic acid (DNA), 8, 17, 19, 22, 23, 30, 33, 39, 41, 60, 64, 71, 90
depression, 14, 92, 93, 94, 95, 111
desipramine, 94
desserts, 58
diet
anticarcinogens and, 10, 63–72
breast cancer and, 57–58
cancer and, 6, 8–11, 49–61, 63–72, 73–80
carcinogens and, 63–72
colorectal cancer and, 58–59
low-risk, 8
policy questions and, 73–80
see also dietary intake data; dietary guidelines; foods; *and specific foods*
Diet, Nutrition, and Cancer, 52, 60
dietary guidelines, 60–61
dietary intake data, 57
DNA, *see* deoxyribonucleic acid; recombinant DNA
Doll, Sir Richard, 55–56
Doyle, Brian, 96
drugs and drug therapy, 6, 11–12, 13, 14, 15, 73, 81, 90, 91, 94, 96, 110
see also chemotherapy
Duesberg, Peter H., 20

E

EDB, *see* ethylene dibromide
eggs, 56, 70
endocrine system, 90
environment, 8, 9, 15, 36, 50, 74

Environmental Protection Agency, 74
enzymes, 25, 26, 71
epidemiology, epidemiologists, and epidemiological studies, 9, 15, 49–61, 63, 64, 68, 69–70, 72
Erickson, Raymond L., 24, 25
esophageal cancer, 61, 68, 70, 74
estragole, 67
ethylene dibromide (EDB), 74
Europe, 53, 104, 105

F

families of cancer patients, psychosocial effects of cancer on, 14, 91–101, 111–114
family history, and cancer, 49, 58
fats, 9, 55–57, 59, 61, 63, 68, 74, 76
fava beans, 68
FDA, *see* Food and Drug Administration
fear, 14, 92, 93, 95, 98–99, 104
Federal Register, 78
fibers, 9, 58, 59, 61, 63, 69, 76
fish, 54, 69, 72
flavonoids, 67, 72
flavorings, 67, 68
Food and Drug Act, 73
Food and Drug Administration (FDA), 73–74, 76, 77–78
food disappearance data, 52
Food, Drug, and Cosmetic Act, 64
  see also Delaney Clause
food safety policy and laws, 11, 72–80
foods
  additives, 9, 10, 63, 73, 74, 75
  browned, 68–69
  burned, 68–69
  cancer and, 9, 51–52, 68–69, 73–80
  contaminants, 9, 10, 68, 73, 74, 77
  cooked, 64, 68, 69, 72
  cured, 61, 65
  fatty, 9
  grilled, 68, 69, 74
  harmful substances in, 10
  labeling of, 77–79
  natural, 63, 64, 65, 74
  pesticides and, 10
  pickled, 61
  processed, 52, 63, 76
  salt-cured, 9
  salt-pickled, 9
  smoked, 61, 68
  spiced, 9
  synthetic, 63
  see also diet; *and specific foods*
forage crops, 65, 67
Frei, Emil, 81, 85, 87, 88, 89
French bread, 69
french fries, 69
fruit flies, 21
fruit jams, 67
fruits, 9, 10, 55, 56, 58, 61, 65, 74, 76
fungi, 66
furocoumarins, 67

G

Gallo, Robert, 42
gas, 68
gastric cancer, 56
gastrointestinal cancer, 55
genes
  abnormal, 5, 7
  active, 33–35, 45–46
  antibody, 41
  cancer and, 5, 6–8, 15, 17–27
  chromosomes and, 8, 18, 19, 23, 39–47
  coding of, 7, 19, 23, 32, 33, 34, 35, 41, 43, 44, 45
  expression of, 44–45, 46
  inactive, 33–35
  mutation of, 8–9, 43
  normal, 7, 33, 37, 43, 45
  proteins and, 6–8, 24–26, 32, 33, 43
  switching of, 36, 37, 41, 43, 45

transforming, 5, 6, 7, 32, 36, 43, 45
viral, 18–21, 29, 30
see also oncogenes; proteins; proto-oncogenes
geneticists and genetic engineering, 6–8, 12, 13, 17–18, 33, 39, 40, 41, 44
GGC (guanine-guanine-cytosine), 34
see also bladder cancer; codon
gin, 104
glutathione, 71
glycine, 34, 35
glycoalkaloids, 68
glycoproteins, 26, 90
grains, 9, 55, 58, 59, 61, 65, 67, 70, 74
Graham, Saxon, 59
Gray, Gregory, 56–57
green vegetables, 69
Greer, David S., 103, 106–116
grief, 92, 95, 100
gross national product, 56
growth factors, 12, 90
GTC (guanine-thymine-cytosine), 34
see also bladder cancer; codon
guanine, 34
Gyromitra esculenta, 66

H

H-*ras*, 32
habits, 78–80
hair follicles, 11, 82
hair loss, 11, 82
hamburgers, 64
Harvey sarcoma virus, 31
Hawaii, 58
Hayward, William S., 23, 42
head and neck cancer, 12, 88–89
Health and Human Services, Department of, 77
Health Care Financing Administration, 106
heart disease, 79
height, 57
Helsing, Knud, 100
Henderson, Maureen, 1
herbal teas, 67
heredity, 9, 17–18, 49
heroin, 104, 106
Hindus, 55
Hodgkin's disease, 86
Holland, Jimmie C., 91–101
honey, 67
Hood, Leroy, 41, 42, 43
hormones, 55, 90
horseradish, 68
hospices
American movement toward, 14, 104–106
assessment of care in, 106–107
compared to hospitals, 104, 107–108, 110, 114
costs of, 114–116
history of, 103–104
home-care, 107–108, 111–116
hospital-based, 107–108, 111–116
intangible elements of care in, 115–116
medical intervention and, 108–110
pain and, 104, 110–111
quality of life and, 111–114
see also hospitals
hospitals, 1, 97, 104, 107–108, 110, 114
see also hospices
Huebner, Robert J., 20–21
human bladder oncogene, 23, 30, 31, 33, 34
Hunter, Tony, 25
hydrazines, 66
hydrogen peroxide, 70
hydroxyl radical, 70

I

imipramine, 94
immune system, 12, 40, 41
immunoglobulin loci, 41

immunology and immunologists, 84, 90
immunotherapy, *see under* chemotherapy
India, 55, 58
individuals, cancer studies on, 57
industrial chemicals and pollutants, 10, 49, 51, 72, 73, 74
infections, 50
infertility, 99
insomnia, 93, 95
insects, 66, 68
interferon, 12, 90
intestinal cancer, 56
intestinal mucosa, 11, 82
intravenous therapy, 108–110
ionizing radiation, 8, 70
Israel, 53–54

J

jams, 76
Japan and Japanese, 53, 54, 56, 58, 68
Jews, 54
John A. Hartford Foundation, 106

K

K-*ras*, 32
Kelly, Kathleen, 45
kidney cancer, 51, 56
kinases, 25, 26
Kirsten sarcoma virus, 31
Klein, George, 41

L

laboratory animals, 59–60, 64, 66, 67, 70, 72
laboratory studies, 6–8, 52, 59–60, 64–65, 68, 69–70
lacto-ovovegetarians, 55
large bowel cancer, 68
laryngeal cancer, 68, 69, 99
Lazarus syndrome, 100
Leder, Philip, 39, 41, 42, 44, 46
Lenoir, Gilbert, 44
lettuce, 65
leukemias, 4, 5, 11, 31, 47, 82, 86, 87, 88
Levinson, Arthur, 25
lifestyle, 9, 50, 51, 56, 79
lip cancer, 56
lipid peroxidation, 71
liver, 5, 69
liver cancer, 5, 70
livestock, 52, 67
London, 103, 104
Lost Chord cancer program, 99
Lubin, Jay, 58
lung cancer, 4, 5, 9, 12, 31, 50, 51, 67, 69, 99
lymph nodes, 84, 87
lymph stream, 6, 87
lymphocytic leukemia, *see* acute lymphocytic leukemia
lymphomas, 32, 40–43, 84, 86, 87
Lyons, Joseph L., 55

M

Marcu, Kenneth, 42, 43
Marks, Paul A., 1, 6, 12, 15
Martin, G. Steven, 20
Martin-Zanca, Dionisio, 35
mastectomy, 99
mayonnaise, 76
McClintock, Barbara, 8
meats, 9, 10, 55, 56, 58, 66, 68, 69, 70, 72, 74, 75
medical staffs, of cancer patients, psychosocial effects of cancer on, 14, 91–101, 111–114
Medicare, 106, 107, 115
medicine, *see* drugs; chemotherapy; hospices; hospitals; surgery; *and specific medicines*
melanomas, 4
meningeal leukemia, 85–86
meninges, 85

6-mercaptopurine, 84
Merrill, Richard, 73, 74, 75–77
metastases, 6, 13, 87
methotrexate, 84
migrants, 50, 53–54
milk, 54, 66
Miller, Anthony B., 49, 57, 59
minerals, 10, 70
see also specific minerals
mitosis, 45
molds, 64, 65, 74
molecular biology and biologists, 1, 6, 7, 8, 12, 15, 18, 26, 29, 30, 32, 89, 91
see also biology and biologists
monkey retrovirus, *see* v-*sis*
monoclonal antibodies, 12
see also antibodies and antibiotics
Mormons, 55
mortality and mortality rates, 4, 100
mos genes, 22
Moulding, Christopher, 44
mouse plasmacytoma, 40
mouth cancer, 68
Mullan, Fitzhugh, 98–99
Multiple Risk Factor Intervention Trial, 79
Murphy, William, 44
mushrooms, 66
mustard, 68
mutagenicity tests, 64, 66
mutagens and mutagenesis, 10, 19, 20, 23, 40, 60, 63–64, 75
myc genes, 20, 23, 31–32, 37, 42–47

N

N-*ras*, 32
narcotics, 106, 110
National Cancer Chemotherapy Program, 83
National Cancer Institute (NCI), 72, 82, 83, 91
National Heart, Lung, and Blood Institute, 79
National Hospice Study, 106, 109, 111, 114
National Research Council, 52, 60–61
nausea, 11, 82, 86, 95
NCI, *see* National Cancer Institute
neck cancer, *see* head and neck cancer
Neel, Benjamin G., 23
New Guinea, 40
New York, 58
nitrates, nitrites, and *N*-nitroso compounds, 65–66, 70, 71
NMR, *see* nuclear magnetic resonance
nortriptyline, 94
Norway, 58
nuclear magnetic resonance (NMR), 13
nucleotides, 23, 31, 33, 45
nutrients, 9, 10, 57, 59, 63, 78
nutrition, 6, 55, 78–79
nuts, 10

O

occupational safety, 77
oils, 56
oncogenes
cancer and, 6–8, 12, 15, 18–26, 29–37, 39–47, 90
cells and, 20–26
discovery of, 8, 15
human, 18
human bladder, 31, 33, 35
mutation of, 34, 35, 36, 40
proteins and, 6–8, 12, 20, 22–26, 29–37, 90
see also genes; proteins; proto-oncogenes
oncology and oncologists, 96
oral cancer, 4
ovarian cancer, 4, 56, 68
oxygen, oxidants, and oxidation, 70–71

P

p21, 32

PAHs, *see* polynuclear aromatic hydrocarbons
pain, 104, 110, 111
pancreatic cancer, 4, 5, 51, 56, 68
Pap smear, 12
Parsis, 55
parsley, 67
parsnips, 67
patients, psychosocial effects of cancer on, 13–14, 91–101, 110, 111–114
peanut butter, 65
peanuts, 64, 65, 75
pecans, 65
pentosan fraction, 58
periwinkle, 85
personal autonomy, 77–78
pesticides, 10, 63, 66–68, 71, 74
pharmacology, 84, 89
pharyngeal cancer, 68
Phillips, Roland, 55
physicians, of cancer patients, psychosocial effects of cancer on, 96
phosphate ions, 25
phosphoproteins, 24
phosphorylation, 25, 26
Pierotti, Marco A., 35
piperine, 67
pistachios, 65
plant chemicals and plant toxins, 66–68, 71
platinum, 89
polio, 15
pollutants, 49, 51
polynuclear aromatic hydrocarbons (PAHs), 68
pork, 58
potatoes, 54, 68, 75
Potter, Huntington, 44
Pott, Percival, 50
pp60v-*src* genes, 24
prednisone, 84, 85
pregnancy, 58
promoters, 60
prostate cancer, 4, 5
proteins
  animal, 55, 56, 57
  cancer and, 6–8, 12, 18, 63, 68, 90
  cells and, 18, 19, 20, 24–26, 43–44, 71
  genes and, 6–8, 24–26, 32, 33, 43
  oncogenes and, 6–8, 12, 20, 22–26, 29–37, 90
  synthesis of, 20, 33
  viruses and, 19–20
  see also amino acids; oncogenes; proto-oncogenes
proto-oncogenes, 21–23, 29–35, 41
  see also genes; oncogenes; proteins
psoralen, 67
psychiatric disorders, *see* psychosocial effects of cancer
psychological effects of cancer, *see* psychosocial effects of cancer
Psychosocial Collaborative Oncology Group, 93, 94
psychosocial effects, of cancer, 6, 13–14, 91–101, 110, 111–114
psychotropic drugs, 14, 94
Punjabis, 58
pyrrolizidine alkaloids, 67

Q

quercetin, 67

R

race, 49
radiation and radiation therapy, 6, 7, 8, 13, 14, 15, 19, 21, 23, 30, 70, 81–82, 87, 88, 97, 98
  see also chemotherapy
radishes, 65
ras genes, 20, 22, 31, 32, 36, 37, 43
rat sarcoma virus, 31
Reach for Recovery cancer program, 99
recombinant DNA, 8

rectal cancer, 4, 5, 53, 56, 59
red wine, 67
Reddy, E. Premkumar, 35
religious groups, 55
renal cancer, 56
relapses, unexpected, 85–86
reproductive organs, 14
research laboratories, 1
retroviruses, 19–23, 29, 30, 32, 35, 43
see also viruses
rhubarb, 65, 68
ribonucleic acid (RNA), 19, 33
rice, 54
Risk Assessment in the Federal Government, 64
RNA, *see* ribonucleic acid
Robert Wood Johnson Foundation, 106
roughage, 58
Rous, Francis Peyton, 18, 19
Rous sarcoma virus, 18, 19, 20, 24
Rowland, Julia, 98

S

saccharin, 76, 78
safrole, 67
Santos, Eugenio, 35
sarcomas, 18, 19, 20
sarsaparilla root beer, 67
sassafras, 67
Saunders, Cicely, 103–104, 106
Scandinavia, 58
Schreiber, Steven, 96
Scolnick, Edward M., 22
Scotch, 68
scrotal cancer, 50
seafood, 70
Sefton, Bartholomew M., 25
selenium, 10, 70, 71
see also minerals
serine, 25
serum cholesterol, 79
Seventh Day Adventists, 55, 58
sex, 55
Shih, Chiaho, 30
skin cancer, 4, 70
skin rashes, 67
smallpox, 15
smoking, *see* cigarette smoking
social effects of cancer, *see* psychosocial effects of cancer
socioeconomic status, 55, 56
soft drinks, 79
solanine, 68
spinach, 65
spinal cord, 85
spinal fluid, 86
spontaneous carcinogenesis, 48–49
see also carcinogens and carcinogenesis
src genes, 20, 21, 24, 25, 26
Stehelin, Dominique, 21
sterigmatocystin, 65
Stewart, Timothy, 44
Stiles, Charles, 45
stomach cancer, 5, 56, 61, 70, 74
stress, 14, 92, 93, 95, 96
sugars, 56, 69, 104
Sugimura, Takashi, 68–69
suicide, 96, 100
superoxide, 70
surgery, 13, 15, 81–82, 87, 88, 91, 97, 99
survivors and survival rates, of cancer, 1, 2, 3, 12–13, 84, 86, 87, 91, 92, 97–98, 100
Szklo, Moyses, 100

T

TAT (thymine-adenine-thymine), 33
see also codon
Taub, Rebecca, 44
tarragon, 67
Tax Equity and Fiscal Responsibility Act (TEFRA), 105, 114
tea, 55, 67, 68, 75
teratogens, 66, 68

testicular cancer, 56, 86
therapeutic nihilism, 94–95
threonine, 25
thymine, 33, 35
  see also TAT
toast, 64, 69
tobacco, 4, 6, 55, 66
tocopherol, *see* vitamin E
Todaro, George J., 20–21
toxicity, 11, 12, 63, 68, 70, 71, 82, 83, 84, 89, 90
toxicology, 66, 84
toxins, 64, 65, 67, 71, 74
tree nuts, 65
tricyclic antidepressants, 94
tumors and tumorigenesis, 5, 8, 12–13, 18–19, 20, 25, 26, 30, 31, 35, 36, 40, 47, 59, 60, 66, 70, 81, 82–84, 87, 90
  see also carcinogens and carcinogenesis
tyrosine, 25

U

ultraviolet radiation, 8
Umbrelliferae family, 67
United Kingdom, 56, 104
United States, 5, 12, 50, 53, 56, 61, 64, 65, 67, 78, 79, 88, 105
U.S. Congress, 14, 76, 83, 105, 106
U.S. government, 10, 77
uric acid, 71
uterine cancer, 4, 5, 52, 56

V

v-*myc*, 21
v-*sis*, 25
v-*src*, 21, 24
vaccines, 15
valine, 34, 35
Vande Woude, George F., 22
Varmus, Harold E., 21, 25
vegetable oil, 70
vegetables, 9, 10, 55, 56, 58, 59, 61, 65, 74, 75, 76
  see also cruciferous vegetables; green vegetables; vegetarians; yellow vegetables; *and specific vegetables*
vegetarians, 55
vincristine, 85
vinegar, 67
virologists and virology, 18–19
viruses, 7, 8, 9, 18, 24, 29, 30, 31, 40, 46, 49, 50, 70, 90
  see also retroviruses
vitamin A, 10, 69, 71
vitamin C, 70, 71
vitamin E, 70, 71
vitamins, 69–70
  see also specific vitamins
vomiting, 11, 82, 86, 95

W

walnuts, 65
water, 70
weight, 57, 58, 77, 79
Weinberg, Robert A., 26, 30, 33, 34, 46
Weissmann, Charles, 20
wheat, whole, 58
whiskey, 68
whites, 3, 53
Wigler, Michael, 30, 33, 34
Wilms' tumor, 88
World War II, 50, 51

X

X rays, 13, 108, 109

Y

yeast, 21
yellow vegetables, 69
Yunis, Jorge, 39